PILATES

FOR EVERY BODY

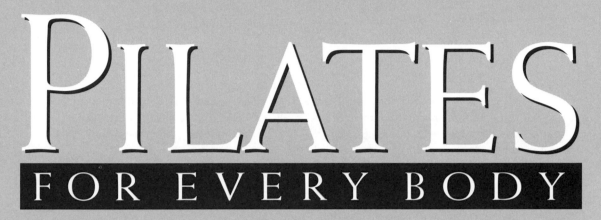

PILATES
FOR EVERY BODY

Strengthen, Lengthen, and Tone—With This
Complete 3-Week Body Makeover

DENISE AUSTIN

STAR OF *THE DAILY WORKOUT* AND *FIT & LITE*, LIFETIME TELEVISION

RODALE

Notice

The information here is designed to help you make decisions regarding your fitness and exercise program. It is not intended as a substitute for professional fitness and medical advice. As with all exercise programs, you should seek your doctor's approval before you begin.

© 2002 by Denise Austin

First published 2002
First published in paperback 2003

Printed in the United States of America
Rodale Inc. makes every effort to use acid-free ∞, recycled paper ♻.

Cover design by Christopher Rhoads
Interior design by Carol Angstadt
Cover photographs by Hilmar (front) and Charles Bush (spine)
Interior photographs by Mary Noble Ours
Illustrations by Karen Kuchar

Library of Congress Cataloging-in-Publication Data

Austin, Denise.
  Pilates for every body : strengthen, lengthen, and tone—with this complete 3-week body makeover / by Denise Austin.
      p.   cm.
  Includes index.
  ISBN 1–57954–613–7 hardcover
  ISBN 1–57954–772–9 paperback
  1. Pilates method.   I. Title.
  RA781 .A875   2002
  613.7'1—dc21   2002005141

Distributed to the book trade by St. Martin's Press

  4 6 8 10 9 7 5 3   hardcover
     6 8 10 9 7 5   paperback

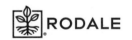

RODALE®

WE **INSPIRE** AND **ENABLE** PEOPLE TO IMPROVE
THEIR LIVES AND THE WORLD AROUND THEM

FOR MORE OF OUR PRODUCTS
WWW.RODALESTORE.COM
(800) 848-4735

To my dear husband, Jeff, who always puts our family first. And to my true joys in life, my girls, Kelly and Katie.

Contents

Denise-eology . . .

"Body shaping . . . body sculpting . . . body lengthening . . . body balancing—not body building."

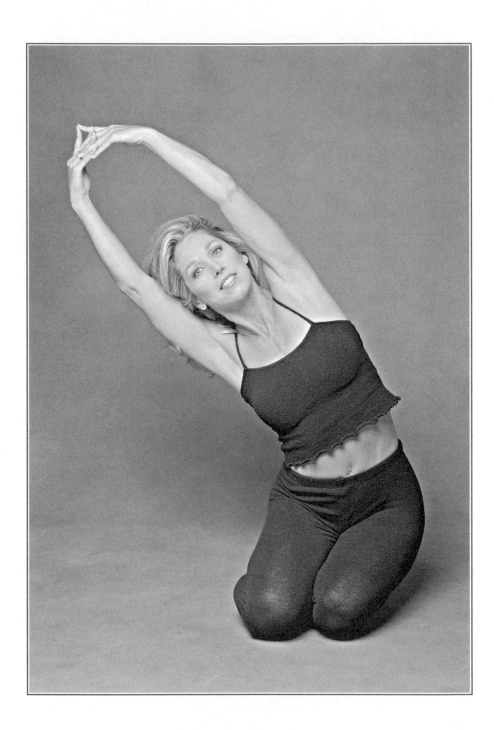

Acknowledgments

When it comes to thanking people, I always think first of Mom. She passed away last year, and a day doesn't go by without me thinking of her. Mom, I miss you so much. You were so dedicated to us five kids. You gave us each other, something for which I'll always be grateful. We're so close, thanks to you and your fun attitude. I love you.

Dad, thank you for teaching me to be strong.

To my sweet husband, Jeff, for always being so loving, supportive, and funny. We've been married 18 years, and I still can't get enough of you. Thanks for being such a wonderful husband and a great dad to our precious girls, Kelly and Katie. I love our family and life together.

I want to thank all the people at Rodale for making this book happen, especially Tami Booth, Elizabeth Crow, Sharon Faelten, and Carol Angstadt.

A huge thanks to Alisa Bauman, who truly made this book happen—and on time. Thank you, you were great.

Special thanks to Michael Broussard and Jan Miller, my literary agents. I love you guys.

There are so many people to thank, especially my great bunch of friends that are always there for me. Thanks from the bottom of my heart.

Denise Austin

Denise Austin

Part

1

WHAT **Pilates** CAN
DO FOR YOU

The POWER behind PILATES

As a health and fitness professional for 25 years, I have taught just about every form of exercise, including strength training, aerobics, and yoga. I firmly believe that regular exercise is the best form of preventive medicine. Great for you both mentally and physically, regular exercise helps you to feel good about yourself. And that's what it's all about—being healthy *and* happy!

Of all the forms of exercise I've taught, Pilates is one of my favorites. I love Pilates because it helps condition the body without punishing the body. Now that I'm 45 years old, that's important to me.

Invented by gymnast Joseph H. Pilates (pronounced puh-*lah*-teez) more than 80 years ago, the Pilates method involves a series of exercises that place intense concentration on your abdominal muscles, particularly the deepest layer of muscles in your abdomen. Besides helping you to form a beautiful flat tummy, strong abdominal muscles will improve your balance and coordination as well as help you perform other types of exercise with more ease.

In addition to firming your abdominals, Pilates also helps strengthen and stretch the entire body from head to toe, helping you to stand taller. This unique system will create long, lean, toned muscles similar to the muscles of a dancer.

The Pilates method combines these exercises with mental concentration and breath-work. The result is a mind-body fitness program that not only helps you create your best body ever but also helps you feel mentally and emotionally balanced, calm, and refreshed.

Pilates for Every Body is a complete Pilates program. You will be focusing on the *total* body: the abs and back, the upper body (arms and shoulders), plus the lower body (hips, buns, and legs). You'll see and feel the results in just 10 sessions.

I've added my own unique twist to Pilates. My approach is more than a series of body moves—it can be customized to individual needs. I've included a number of routines from which you can choose. Some of these routines will help you target particular trouble spots, such as the hips, thighs, and buns. Others will help you address particular health concerns, such as a bad back. Some are designed for on-the-go people with little time to exercise, whereas others offer a more complete, vigorous workout.

I've also included numerous variations on exercises—from beginner level to more challenging. Because many exercises can be done from a seated or reclining position, they can be performed by people who are overweight or have bad knees and therefore can't take jarring exercise like jogging. No matter what your fitness level, health background, or time constraints, you'll find a routine that helps you build a lean, strong, balanced body in as little as 3 weeks.

The Story of Pilates

Contrary to what many people assume, the Pilates method is not new. Joseph Pilates first developed the Pilates method of body conditioning to help rehabilitate bed-bound patients at a hospital in England where he worked as a nurse during World War I. To enable patients to regain

"Pilates can help you go from
fat to flab-free at any age."

strength, Pilates attached springs to their mattresses for them to pull and push against for resistance.

When Joseph Pilates moved to New York City in the 1920s, he brought the conditioning method he'd perfected with him. At first, injured dancers would come to Pilates for help. He put them through a series of exercises on a machine he called the Reformer. This bedlike apparatus featured a horizontal sliding platform with springs that could be adjusted to allow for differing levels of resistance.

Some of Pilates' first clients included the famed dancer, teacher, and choreographer Martha Graham and renowned choreographer George Balanchine. Soon, dancers all over New York City were knocking on Joseph Pilates' door. Even one of my closest friends and colleagues Cal Pozo, then a Broadway dancer, went to Pilates for help after he injured his hip while dancing in the musical *West Side Story* in the late 1950s.

I met Cal many years later, in 1988, when he helped me choreograph one of my first exercise videos. He's been a mentor to me ever since, and his expertise in Pilates encouraged me to create my *Mat Workout Based on the Work of J. H. Pilates* and *Pilates for Every Body* videos.

Because Joseph Pilates wanted to help as many people as he could, in the 1960s he developed a series of exercises that could be performed on mats, without any machines, and accomplish the same benefits of improved body mechanics; lean, supple muscles; and overall body conditioning. Over the years, Pilates' mat method spread, and now Hollywood celebrities such as Madonna, Sharon Stone, and Julia Roberts and professional athletes, including professional football players such as the San Francisco 49ers, are doing Pilates.

As more and more people tried the Pilates method, word continued to spread. Soon, Pilates studios began popping up all over the country, in big cities and small towns, making the method accessible not only to the rich and famous, but to everyone. Today, the Pilates method is used all over the world by a diverse number of people, including spa goers, fitness enthusiasts, athletes, and those in the performing arts.

To me, that's the most exciting aspect of Pilates. It doesn't matter who you are—athlete or couch potato, toned or flabby, man or woman, young or old—you can do it.

Every body can benefit. That's why I've included so many different routines in this book. Each routine helps address a specific goal, so even each reader can use this book for different reasons at different times.

You can choose the routine that best fits your needs right now, and later on choose a different routine if and when needed. With *Pilates for Every Body*, you will always have the variety you need to stay motivated!

Your Abs Are Your "Powerhouse"

The secret to the success of Pilates doesn't lie in the actual Pilates moves. Many of them look no different than your basic situp, crunch, or yoga pose. The real key lies in what we call the powerhouse—your abdomen, your center, the *core* of your body.

Pilates works the deepest layer of your abdominal muscles to completely realign and reshape your body. Unlike weight lifting, which focuses on one muscle at a time, Pilates works your body as a unit, starting with your core and lengthening upward and outward. During weight lifting and even during a stomach crunch, you strengthen as you shorten your muscles, essentially bringing the ends of each muscle closer together. During Pilates moves, you work your muscles through a fuller range of motion. You strengthen as you lengthen the muscle, so the ends of the muscles are farther apart, not contracted. This combination of stretching and strengthening helps you create a lean, toned body, like a dancer's.

Four muscles make up your abdominals: the rectus abdominis, the internal and external obliques, and the transverse abdominis. Your rectus abdominis forms the "six-pack," the front of your abs that reaches vertically from your sternum to your pelvic bone. Many people—even those who do daily crunches—have a weak spot at the bottom of their rectus abdominis, below the navel. That's where most tummies tend to bulge. My Pilates exercises will address that weak spot and zero in right where you need it.

Pilates will also target your internal and external obliques, the abdominal muscles that form your waist along the sides of your abdomen, and your transverse abdominis, a deep abdominal muscle not worked

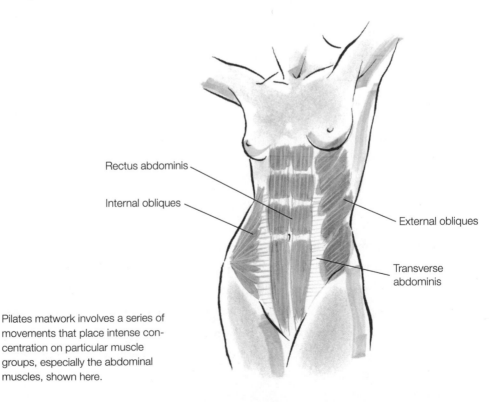

Rectus abdominis

Internal obliques

External obliques

Transverse abdominis

Pilates matwork involves a series of movements that place intense concentration on particular muscle groups, especially the abdominal muscles, shown here.

in many other forms of abdominal exercise. Your transverse abdominis supports your back and holds in your belly. A strong transverse abdominis is the key to good posture, a pain-free back, and a flat tummy.

Pilates will also strengthen and stretch your erector spinae, the muscles along your spine that hold your spinal column straight and upright. It will keep your entire torso strong and supple from front to back.

All of that works together to create a strong core, giving you more balance, coordination, strength, and flexibility. We call this the powerhouse because, truly, that's where you find your power. Pilates is part explosive (short burst) power and part endurance, the combination of which gives you both strength and grace.

How I've Benefited from Pilates

Pilates has brought my sports and fitness career full circle. I started training in gymnastics at the age of 12 and practiced 4 to 5 hours a day, competing and even earning a full athletic scholarship to college. It was my life. As I look back on my gymnastics training some 30 years ago, I realize that Pilates-like exercises were a part of our warmup and conditioning. (Joseph Pilates was also a gymnast.) Moves like V-sits (called the teaser in Pilates) and T-stands prepare gymnasts to do kip-ups on the uneven bars and handstands on the balance beam. But don't worry, I won't expect you to do flips, somersaults, or cartwheels!

I began doing Pilates-type exercises during the early 1990s and soon realized that Pilates was fast becoming one of my secrets to staying young and fit.

In my personal fitness plan, I began to do Pilates three times a week, fitting my sessions in after my morning power walk. I've also altered some of my regular toning moves to make them more Pilates-esque. The combined approach allowed me to effectively condition my entire body while simultaneously feeling the lengthening of my muscles.

The results were undeniable. Various people, including my husband, told me that my legs looked leaner. Though my abs have always been my forte, Pilates helped me to keep them flat and strong, even after having two babies. At 5 feet 4 inches tall, I've always wanted extra height, and I definitely didn't want to shrink as I aged. Pilates helped me to stand taller, making me feel as though I'm 5-foot-6.

Discovering Pilates during my late thirties was a blessing. I realized I needed a simpler, gentler way to stay in shape without any bouncing or jarring to my joints.

The smooth, gentle, flowing movement of Pilates provided that answer. Pilates helps me balance my cardio workouts and build strong, flexible muscles. While I still walk/run and lift weights, Pilates offers me a combined toning and stretching workout, helping me to create a more balanced body from the inside out.

Even on my busiest of days, I do a little Pilates, even if it's just 5 or 10 minutes. My mini-workouts help me to feel stretched and toned from head to toe. They also help keep my spine strong and healthy, another great benefit of Pilates.

What My Fans Tell Me

After studying with some of the top master trainers at the time, I began incorporating Pilates into my *Fit & Lite* show on Lifetime TV, combining the Pilates moves with my own total-body toning exercises and cardio routines.

Viewers loved it. I received thousands of letters from people telling me how much they enjoyed and benefited from the show. *Fit & Lite* soon became the number one fitness show on television, and it still is today.

I was so excited by my results and the positive feedback from the *Fit & Lite* show that in 2000, I came out with my *Mat Workout Based on the Work of J. H. Pilates* video, and it became the top-selling exercise video in the nation. I soon began receiving wonderful e-mails and letters from so many people, telling me how my Pilates workouts were helping them.

These excited women and men told me they felt stronger and leaner and had no more back problems. Plus they felt more balanced and co-ordinated. Pilates had completely changed the shape of their bodies. They had lost inches in their waistline and thighs. Some had grown as much as an inch taller! One marathon runner told me that only Pilates—and not all those miles on the road—transformed her body, flattened her tummy, and lifted her buns.

Here's what some people had to say:

"I do your Pilates video and *Fit & Lite* show every day if possible," says Tammy, age 40. "I have gone from a size 18 to a size 12. I feel so much better, but I'm not through. I will get even slimmer, thanks to you."

Diane, a college student about to be married, wrote to say, "I do your *Pilates Mat Workout* and *Power Yoga Plus* videos every other day. The 20-minute sessions help me to alleviate the stress of everyday life. Last semester I got a 4.0 *and* a healthy body! I really do feel taller and leaner, and for the first time in my life I have muscle tone and the washboard stomach that I've always wanted. I am now planning my wedding, and I am going to look great in my dress!"

Pilates also helped Merlinda Seis, 29, a hairdresser in Colorado Springs, get her weight under control. "Last March I got on the scale and didn't like the number I saw—160 pounds! I bought your *Pilates Mat Workout* video, and 9 months later I was down to 144 pounds," says Merlinda. "Thank you for working out with me at home. I really enjoy it!"

Denise-eology . . .

"Take a few minutes each day to relax. It's easy and takes barely any time. Close your eyes, take a few deep breaths, and just let go."

Men and women alike see amazing results. "I first discovered Pilates on your *Fit & Lite* show," says Erin R. Myers, 24, a financial representative in Baltimore. "It has really increased my abdominal strength—much more than doing crunches ever did. You have even inspired my husband, a Marine, to try Pilates. He was so impressed by the results that he showed the moves to some other Marines in his squad."

Combining Pilates with regular cardio exercise makes it a total conditioning program, with mind-body benefits. "A year and a half ago, I was 75 pounds over my goal weight. I saw a picture of myself and finally realized how out of control my life had become," says Kelly Brandt, 30, of O'Fallen, Montana. "For my daily routine, I now wake up each morning and do the Pilates moves on your *Fit & Lite* show. Then I do 30 minutes of some type of cardio exercise. Every other evening, I do 20 minutes of your Pilates video. I am now at my goal weight and have never felt better. I feel so invigorated after doing the Pilates moves. I feel stronger, leaner, and full of energy when I'm done. I can truly say that you have changed my life. I would definitely recommend Pilates to anyone who wants to feel better physically *and* mentally."

Many viewers report that Pilates worked in ways that other forms of exercise did not. "The Pilates method is the only exercise I've done where I actually achieved results," says Charyl Cammarota, 46, a legal secretary in Collingswood, New Jersey. "My tummy has always been a problem area. It was never flat, even after I lost 35 pounds. But your Pilates video and *Fit & Lite* show have worked wonders. My tummy has reduced considerably. Also, when I finish the exercises, I *feel* skinny and lean. I'm more alert and have more energy and stamina. (I almost never get midafternoon slumps anymore.) My blood pressure and cholesterol are under control. In fact, during my yearly checkup a few weeks ago, my gynecologist told me that I was in better health and shape than most women my age!"

The beauty of Pilates is its versatility—people can benefit in diverse ways. Numerous new moms wrote to say that Pilates helped to flatten their tummies and lose their "baby weight." One fan wrote to tell me that building her core strength with Pilates had helped her become a better dancer and cheerleader. Another wrote to tell me that Pilates helped her stay fit after she developed arthritis in her knees, hips, and shoulders and could no longer do high-impact aerobics. And a hard-core power lifter told me that Pilates helped him recover faster after hard gym workouts.

Those letters and the people I've met convinced me to write this book, to share this amazing method with so many others. I want to share with you everything about Pilates so you can be fit and stay fabulous forever.

I know Pilates works for every body, based on feedback not only from my fans but also from my family and friends. For example, I introduced Pilates to my older sister Kristine, who was immediately drawn to the exercises because they reminded her of the types of exercises she used to do in her ballet classes during childhood.

My sister Donna, whom I always prod to exercise, has also benefited from doing my Pilates workouts. My sister Anne, who has had all three of her children by cesarean section, really needed to firm and strengthen her lower tummy. I convinced her to do the 10-Minute Advanced Abdominal Routine (in part 3 of this book). She does it almost every day, and it shows on her flat tummy.

My brother, Michael, has also tried a few moves to keep his back flexible for his job as a home builder. Finally, my husband, Jeff, sometimes joins me for my Pilates session at home. The T-stands in particular have helped him to streamline his waistline and sport six-pack abs at age 50!

Every Body Benefits from Pilates

Possibly one of the most exciting aspects of Pilates is that anyone can do it, and everyone can achieve amazing results. Because there's no bouncing, jarring, or stress to your body, Pilates offers the ideal form of exercise for people who, because of joint pain or muscle weakness, shy away from exercise.

"There is nothing more rewarding than taking care of yourself."

It's also convenient. Whether you follow this book or my *Pilates for Every Body* video, you won't need any heavy, expensive equipment, and you can do Pilates anywhere, anytime. Some of the routines in this book take less than 10 minutes, making Pilates the perfect form of exercise for anyone who finds there's not enough time in the day for exercise. You have 10 minutes to strengthen your abs and back, don't you? You'll start to see and feel results in as few as 10 sessions.

To sum up, here are just some of the many ways you'll benefit from doing Pilates regularly.

A healthy, supple spine. Pilates gives more support to your spine, creating space between between each vertebra. That extra space not only makes you appear taller, it also creates more mobility, transforming your spine from a stiff rod into a supple string of pearls. This new suppleness prevents degenerative spinal problems, such as slipped disks. It also helps you move with more grace and ease.

Better balance, more coordination. In your forties, balance starts to deteriorate as your muscles weaken and your nerve receptors lose sensitivity. Pilates reverses this aging process by stabilizing your core. Pilates works small, deep muscles needed to keep your body steady when walking and your spine both supple and strong.

Less pain and stiffness. If you suffer from osteoarthritis pain, you'll find that lengthening your body through Pilates will help soothe the soreness. Appropriate exercise is vital to managing arthritis, because it increases flexibility for stretches and reduces pain and fatigue. Stretching helps pump vital nutrients to your muscles and tendons, which help keep them healthy and minimize your risk of injury. It also stimulates the production of joint lubricants (synovial fluid) and pre-

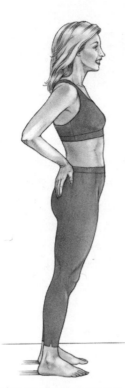

Many of us compensate for weak abdominals and tight back muscles by thrusting the hips forward, arching the lower back, and pouching out the tummy. This weakens and stretches the lower abs, important muscles needed to flatten your belly. Your shoulders, in turn, respond to weak abs by slumping forward.

Pilates reverses bad posture by strengthening your lower belly, which pulls your pelvis back into position. That, in turn, lifts your hip flexors, lengthens the fronts of your thighs, and reduces the arch in your back. As you strengthen your powerhouse, all of these beneficial changes will occur naturally. You'll find yourself standing taller, without having to constantly remind yourself to stop slouching.

vents adhesions. As circulation increases, your legs, back, neck, and shoulders loosen up, relieving aches and stiffness. One of my friends, who is 57, thought her arthritis would never improve. Then she tried my Pilates routines, and her joint pain disappeared!

Pilates also leads to subtle posture improvements, which will also eliminate tension, driving away headaches, backaches, neck aches, and other aches and pains.

Kinder, gentler conditioning. If you're out of shape, Pilates provides a wonderful way to ease into any kind of fitness plan. Pilates puts no stress on your joints and no wear and tear on your ligaments and cartilage around your joints, especially your knee and shoulder joints. It conditions your muscles in a balanced way and increases your self-awareness by drawing your focus inward. In reality, Pilates is very rehabilitative. It's almost like going to physical therapy sessions. In fact, unlike other forms of exercise, you can safely do Pilates every day without overstressing your muscles or joints. To see results, however, you need to do Pilates only three times a week. But you have to be consistent. That's the key.

Improved mental outlook and increased motivation. Pilates also benefits your emotional health. The smooth, steady movements quiet your mind and soothe your nervous system. As you lengthen and strengthen your muscles, you'll improve your circulation and whisk tension away. Each workout will leave you feeling calm, balanced, and rejuvenated. Focus on letting the tension go, and you'll be on the path to a healthier body inside and out.

Faster return to prepregnancy figure. Many women who have given birth ask me how I got my lower tummy so flat after I had my two kids. I show them three simple Pilates moves—the crisscross (page 78), the double-leg stretch (page 76), and the frog (page 174). The women do the moves, and they work. It doesn't take that much time, but if you do a few moves on a regular basis, you will see results. Muscles have a beautiful memory. They will bounce back with a just little toning.

My Pilates PRIMER

Every Pilates movement—when done correctly—starts in your core (abdomen), stays in your core, and ends in your core. A strong core:

- Allows a gymnast to hold a handstand and a yogi to hold a headstand
- Allows the martial artist to kick through a board and a dancer to leap into the air
- Puts more oomph in your tennis swing, more speed to your run, and more control in your ski slalom
- Creates power in your midsection and shrinks middle-age spread, helping you to accomplish goals you never before dreamed possible

That's why it's so important that you learn how to move from your core before you attempt any Pilates routine. If you lose the core emphasis, you lose many of the benefits of Pilates.

To understand what I'm talking about, try this simple exercise, which I call "zipping up your abs":

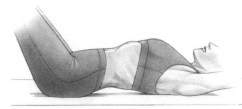 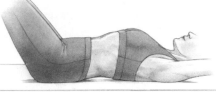

Lie back on the floor, with your knees bent, your flat feet on the floor, and your back slightly arched, as shown on the left. Focus on your pelvic area and your lower abdomen, below the belly button. Pull those muscles up and inward, as if you were zipping up a corset. This upward and inward motion will bring your belly button toward your spine as well as lengthen your torso, creating more space between your ribs and hips.

Notice how you've slightly lifted your pelvis and flattened your back but still have a slight neutral curve in your lower back, as shown on the right. Take note of the length in your core. Memorize this sensation.

Imagine that zipper again. Now try to zip yourself up even tighter, lengthening as the imaginary zipper comes up your midsection, almost squeezing yourself taller. This is how you want to feel during every Pilates exercise.

In addition to "zipping up your abs," follow these posture pointers during every Pilates exercise.

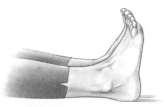 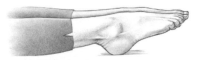

Your feet. Some moves require you to flex your feet, as shown on the left. Others require you to point, or extend them, as shown on the right. When flexing your feet, press through your heels to create length in your body, but keep your toes straight, not curled back toward your shins. When pointing your toes, create length by extending through your big toe, but don't overpoint, or overextend, by curling your toes toward your arches.

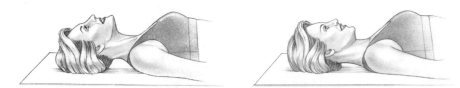

Your neck. Don't arch your neck, as shown on the left. Whether sitting or lying in position to do Pilates, you want a long neck. Concentrate on lengthening through the crown of your head and tuck your chin toward your neck slightly, as shown on the right.

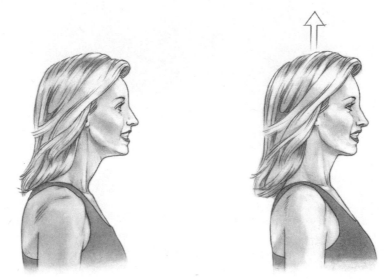

Your head. Don't lead with your chin or allow your shoulders to slouch forward, as shown on the left. Instead, center your head directly above your shoulders, as shown on the right. Your ears should feel aligned with your shoulders. To lengthen your spine, imagine a rod running from the crown of your head through your tailbone.

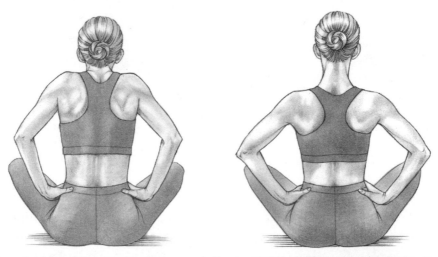

Your shoulders. Many people, when concentrating, hunch their shoulders toward their ears, as shown on the left. This creates neck tension and constricts breathing. You want your shoulders low and drawn back, opening your chest, as shown on the right. Think about bringing your shoulder blades down your back toward your hips. Then, roll your shoulders up and back. You should feel your chest open.

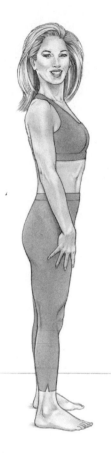

Put it all together. Stand with your feet in the proper position, with the joint between your big and second toes under your knees. Pull your pelvic muscles up and in, flatten your abs toward your spine, lengthen through your ribs, lengthen through your crown, and relax your shoulder blades down and back. Doesn't that feel wonderful? Can you feel the energy this posture creates?

The Principles of Pilates

As you start each Pilates session, it's important to keep these nine principles in mind.

Concentration. To do Pilates moves correctly, you'll need to concentrate on your abs—keeping them pulled in and up—at all times. Think "long" and "lean." Keep your body long by extending through your torso.

Breathing. Because Pilates requires you to press your abs toward your spine, you don't want to allow your lower belly to round and press out as air comes into your lungs. You also don't want that abdominal lock to force you to breathe shallowly. To breathe correctly, you must expand your rib cage, primarily through your midback.

This breathing technique can feel awkward at first, so try it now. Sit up nice and tall. As you inhale, keep your lower abs pressed flat but encourage your ribs to expand outward with your breath, as if you had a hula hoop around your rib cage and were trying to expand your ribs to hold the hoop in place. As you breathe, you should feel a stretch through your ribs and midback. It should feel good!

Breathe in through your nose and out through your mouth. As you exhale, sigh audibly. It will help you relax.

As you move with your breath, you'll automatically breathe more deeply in order to match your inhalations with your body movements. This deep inhaling and exhaling rids your lungs of stale air and fills them with fresh, oxygen-filled air, energizing your entire body. Allow your body to move to its cadence. This will help you stay in the moment, making your Pilates practice meditative.

As you do Pilates, use your breath to draw your mind into the present and whisk the tension out of your body. In every exercise, keep your abs "engaged" and elongate your spine. The instructions for each exercise tell you when to inhale and when to exhale. For now, just remember that you should breathe as you move.

Control. In other fitness pursuits, you may have learned to go through the motions first and perfect your form second. In Pilates, it's the other way around. You learn to control your abs first and then proceed through a series of more progressive movements. At all times, you

Denise-eology . . .
"Energy is found in oxygen.
So breathe deep, nourishing,
energizing breaths!"

"Pilates is my mental filter.
      It filters out any anxieties and
    makes me feel relaxed, energized,
    and fun to be around."

should feel in control of your body. If you don't, you're moving beyond your ability level. Make each movement slow and controlled. Make each movement count.

Center focus. Everything in Pilates starts in your center—your abs and powerhouse—and moves outward. Before every exercise, pay attention to your center, making sure those abdominal muscles are pulled up and in. Eventually, you'll maintain a strong center even while standing in the checkout line at the grocery store, sitting at your desk, driving your car, or watching TV.

Fluidity. Pilates is a fluid series of exercises, with each exercise smoothly leading into the next. You rarely stop to hold a pose. You should feel graceful as you perform these exercises.

Precision. Throughout this book, I offer my Pilates Pointers to help you get an exercise just right, so you benefit fully. Pay attention to all the Pilates Pointers for each move. Just the slightest adjustment can make all of the difference between really feeling a move and not feeling it at all.

Imagination. If you see yourself doing Pilates exercises in your mind, you'll pick them up faster. When I practiced gymnastics, I would imagine myself executing a perfect floor routine. The visualization helped me perform better. Imagine yourself executing perfect exercises, then do them. You'll be amazed at how your imagination can transform your results.

"Don't lose sleep over things you cannot change. Wash away guilt. It's not worth it. Strive for balance of health, fitness, nutrition, and happiness."

Intuition. You may have heard the saying, "Listen to your body." Pilates will teach you to fine-tune that skill. Pay attention to how your body feels in every exercise. If something hurts, don't force yourself through it. You may simply need to fine-tune the exercise. Keep practicing. Eventually, you'll be at one with your body, allowing its intuition to tell you how many repetitions to do and how long to hold a stretch. Some days, you'll feel more flexible and stronger than others. Do the best you can and always listen to your body.

Integration. In Pilates, you work your body as a unit. You'll soon integrate this principle into everyday life. You'll notice that you walk with ease. Rather than only using your legs, you'll use your entire body. This integration will give you a new grace to your movements, and, believe me, people will notice a connection with your "whole body"!

And finally, before getting started, do something simple yet effective. Put a smile on your face.

What You'll Need

Many people think of a machine called the Reformer when they think of Pilates. Typically found in Pilates studios or in Pilates classes offered at health clubs, the machine adds resistance, creating a very effective Pilates workout. However, unless you live in a big city, it may be tough to find fitness clubs that have Reformer machines, and those that offer private lessons on the Reformer can be quite expensive.

The routines in this book simulate exercises performed on the Reformer and use the same muscles, at a fraction of the cost. You'll need only a comfortable surface to lie on—such as an exercise mat (available wherever sporting goods are sold), a thick towel, or a carpeted floor. For some of the exercises, you may need a pillow or cushion, a chair, a large exercise ball (sometimes called a resistance ball or a stability ball), elastic exercise bands, or a set of light dumbbells (2 to 5 pounds each for most women or 8 to 10 pounds each for stronger women and for men).

You don't even need fancy exercise clothes or shoes. Just wear clothing that feels comfortable and allows you to move easily. You can even do Pilates barefoot, if that's your choice. I do recommend wearing shoes, however, for routines that require hand weights, just in case you drop one on your foot.

How to Use This Book

Throughout the next three parts of this book, I offer numerous Pilates routines from which to choose. In some of these routines, I've added a touch of yoga, ballet, and strength training—all with a Pilates emphasis. No matter which routine or routines you select, they provide total-body sculpting and conditioning.

Denise-eology . . .

"Aging is 70 percent lifestyle.
To stay young, eat right,
exercise regularly, and keep
a positive attitude."

In part 2, The Core Movements, I offer three different Pilates routines: the Beginner Pilates Program, the Complete Pilates Program, and a Warmup and Cooldown Program. The Beginner Pilates Program is a great way to start if you're out of shape or overweight, have recently had a baby, or experience chronic pain, such as a bad back or arthritis. After doing the routines in the Beginner Pilates Program for 3 weeks or more, you'll be ready for the Complete Pilates Program, an intermediate routine. If you've been practicing yoga or have done my *Power Yoga Plus* video, my *Mat Workout Based on the Work of J. H. Pilates* video, or my *Pilates for Every Body* video, you may be strong and flexible enough to skip the Beginner Pilates Program and start with the Complete Pilates Program. Use the Warmup and Cooldown Program before or after your Pilates routine of choice or after the cardio exercise regimens suggested in part 4.

Anytime, Anywhere

All you need to do Pilates is 4 feet of floor space—sometimes even less. So you can do Pilates almost anywhere—on your bedroom floor, in your office at work, or even in a small hotel room when you travel. I find myself doing Pilates in the strangest of places. For example, while driving in the car or while standing in line, I concentrate on "zipping up my abs."

Pilates workouts are meant to be smooth and soothing, so eliminate distractions before you start. Unless you're watching my *Pilates for Every Body* video or following my *Fit & Lite* program on Lifetime Television, turn off the TV. Put on some soft music. Clear your mind of your thoughts.

This isn't easy, I know. We are all so busy that our minds race constantly. Try to keep your mind in the moment by concentrating on your breathing. If your mind returns to thoughts of your grocery list, push it aside by focusing on your breathing. As you move through the postures, your breathing will draw you to the present.

In part 3, Pick Your Plan, I offer six mini-routines that target specific trouble spots—your abs, your back, your upper body, or your hips, thighs, and buttocks—and accomplish specific goals. Each of these routines takes 10 minutes or less and will help you zero in on specific areas that need improvement.

In part 4, I offer my 3-Week Total Body Makeover. This comprehensive, progressive program combines Pilates with an eating plan, an in-home cardio exercise plan, and a positive-thinking plan. It also includes a diary to help you track your progress. This program will reshape both your body and mind. So it's the ideal way to use this book, if you have time for all the components. After progressing through this 3-week plan, you can choose any of the other plans that you like. For example, you could go on to try the Complete Pilates Program in part 2 and mix and match other routines as you wish.

While many of the exercises in these programs may look easy, you'll quickly see how much strength it takes to hold your body in these positions. Take your time and don't get discouraged, especially if you're a beginner. As you do each move, focus on maintaining proper form and alignment; don't sacrifice form to save a few seconds. Your movements should be smooth and fluid. If you have trouble with a move, don't get frustrated. Keep practicing, and soon you'll develop the strength and flexibility you need. You'll be amazed at how quickly your body will progress from one workout to the next.

After just 10 sessions, Pilates will become a natural part of your life, as it has mine, allowing you to keep a Pilates mental and physical focus everywhere you go and keep that tummy tucked in naturally.

Part

2

THE Core MOVEMENTS

Three Complete
PROGRAMS,
One Primary
EMPHASIS

This section provides you with three complete Pilates routines: the Beginner Pilates Program, the Complete Pilates Program (a more challenging, intermediate routine), and the Warmup and Cooldown Program.

I call these exercises—64 in all—the core movements for two reasons. First, these routines focus on the core exercises first developed by Joseph H. Pilates in the 1920s. (Other routines in this book incorporate some dance, weight lifting, and other moves, giving them a stronger dose of my personal approach.) Second, each and every exercise in the following three routines target your core—your abdominal muscles. As I mentioned in part 1, a strong abdomen helps create a longer, leaner, more balanced and supple body.

Within each series, the movements are performed according to how your body and mind typically respond to exercise. The beginner and complete series, for example, start with gentle, easy stretches then move on to basic strengthening moves that take only a little coordination. The first few exercises in each routine focus on your back, stretching and warming those muscles so that they don't strain when challenged with the next sequence of exercises in the routine. Then you move into poses that work your abs, hip flexors, and thighs, increasing blood circulation and firming and toning those areas. Following those are poses that help loosen your spine. You conclude with tougher poses that require balance and more coordination, as well as strength and flexibility along the sides, front, *and* back of your body.

Every movement we do is for a reason. So do them in order. Though each routine will help you achieve slightly different goals, they all have the same emphasis: building core strength. In every exercise, press your belly button toward your spine as described on page 17 in part 1.

Here's how to determine which program is most appropriate for you, based on the aims of each of the three routines and the ways you can benefit.

The Beginner Pilates Program

If you've never done Pilates until now or you're out of shape, you've recently had a baby, you're overweight, or you have chronic neck, lower back, or joint pain, start with the beginner program, on page 35. I've modified traditional Pilates movements to allow you to strengthen your core and stretch and lengthen key muscles more comfortably than in the intermediate program. In many, I've used aids, such as towels and pillows, to ease strain on your neck. In others, I've simplified the pose— by bending the knees, for example, and allowing you to use your arm

Denise-eology . . .

"You will see results with Pilates.
It is worth it because
you are worth it!"

strength for balance—to make it easier for a beginner to perform the move. While all of the Pilates moves are easy on the joints, the exercises in the Beginner Pilates Program are less demanding and complicated than the moves in the Complete Pilates Program.

The Beginner Pilates Program also includes key exercises to help you get in shape for the Complete Pilates Program.

The beginner routine takes less than 20 minutes to complete. Don't rush—and do the 18 movements in order, as each exercise will prepare your body for the one that comes next. Once you learn the movements, you can follow the "shorthand" version of these routines, for easy reference, to help you move fluidly in the proper sequence. You will find it on page 60, following the fully demonstrated routine.

The Complete Pilates Program

Some of the 36 exercises in this intermediate sequence, on page 63, are easy enough for beginners to tackle, while many others require more coordination, strength, and flexibility. To do all 36 movements in order requires quite a bit of abdominal strength, back flexibility, and overall endurance. You're ready for this sequence if you've done the Beginner Pilates Program for 3 weeks or more, if you've completed my 3-Week Total Body Makeover in part 4 of this book, if you've been practicing power yoga or gone to Pilates classes for a few months, or if you regularly exercise with my *Fit & Lite* television program, my *Mat Workout Based on the Work of J. H. Pilates* video, my *Pilates for Every Body* video, or my *Power Yoga Plus* video workout.

This Pilates sequence provides you with the full breadth of stretching and strengthening moves that you need for a long, lean, supple, strong body from head to toe.

The Complete Pilates Program will take a little more than 30 minutes to complete. As with the Beginner Pilates Program, perform these exercises in the sequence provided. Each movement will prepare your body for the one that comes next. If you lack the time, strength, flexibility, or endurance to perform all 36 moves in one workout, try the shorter 18-movement Beginner Pilates Program instead, then try this again when you feel ready.

Once you learn the movements, you can follow the shorthand version of this program, for quick reference, starting on page 114.

The Warmup and Cooldown Program

The third sequence of the core movements, on page 119, includes my favorite stretches. Use them as a warmup or a cooldown before or after the Beginner Pilates Program or the Complete Pilates Program. You can also use them after any aerobic activities, such as walking, or even after you do a workout with light weights. You can do them any time your body needs to loosen up—for example, to give yourself a break after working at a computer for hours.

The Warmup and Cooldown Program will take a little more than 10 minutes to complete, and it feels wonderful. As with the first two routines, these stretches form a complete sequence. Do them in order, flowing from one stretch into the next. Once you learn the stretches, you can follow the shorthand version of this program, for quick reference, beginning on page 132.

Keys to Pilates Success

With each movement, I've given pointers to help you visualize the exercise, use correct form, and perform the moves safely. Overall, here's what to keep in mind.

Think Quality over Quantity

Doing Pilates correctly requires concentration. The exercises may feel awkward at first, and you may not get every pose right on your first try. Just do your best. It's okay to modify poses by not completing the full range of motion suggested. But never cheat by releasing your abs, allowing them to push outward. Rather, keep pressing your navel toward your spine all the time. That's the key to Pilates success.

Think "Long," Not "High"

When people perform situps, forward bends, or any other stretching or strengthening move, they often try to touch their noses to their knees,

Breathe As You Move

If Pilates is new to you, you may find yourself holding your breath as you concentrate on executing the exercises. Remember to breathe—it will help you to relax.

Your breath will also give you renewed strength to hold a pose just a little longer and make your routines feel meditative. In part 1, I've explained more specifically how to breathe for Pilates. Here are some additional pointers.

• For challenging exercises, I use what I call percussion breathing: Inhale quickly twice and exhale quickly twice. Think in, in, out, out. Inhale and exhale forcefully, making a percussive, audible sound with your breath. Use your entire rib cage to quickly draw in air two times and press out air two times. You'll be amazed how this boosts your endurance, strength, and flexibility. In one particular exercise, the hundred (page 66), I expand on this technique by inhaling five times, and exhaling five times in a percussive fashion. The increased number of breaths helps warm your entire body, readying it for subsequent moves.

• For exercises that require you to sink into a deep stretch, I suggest you breathe deeply to encourage your muscles to relax. Just as deep, cleansing breaths help during childbirth, they also help you sink deeper into a stretch. Inhale deeply, filling up your lungs, and exhale with a sigh.

• For most other exercises, simply breathe normally, bringing the air in through your nose and out through your mouth. Try to match your breathing to your movement, and never hold your breath.

lift their shoulders as high off the floor as possible, or perform some other physical challenge. In Pilates, instead of trying to look impressive, try to lengthen your body. For example, in the Superman (on page 83), instead of raising your hands and feet as high as possible, perform the movement in a way that attempts to elongate your body through your crown, creating as much length in your spine as you can. You won't be able to lift your shoulders as far off the ground, but you'll perform the exercise more effectively.

Denise-eology . . .

"In Pilates, we are creating long, lean-looking muscles . . . not big, bulky muscles."

The BEGINNER Pilates PROGRAM

The Beginner Pilates Program offers the optimal exercise sequence for those who are overweight or out of shape, or who have arthritis, a sore back, or a weak lower belly from a recent pregnancy. (If you're pregnant, talk to your doctor before starting any new exercise program, including Pilates, and don't try any moves on your back after the second trimester.)

If you have arthritis or back pain or have recently been pregnant, my 10-Minute Healthy Back Routine on page 186, in part 3, also targets important muscle groups to help you get and stay healthy.

Unless otherwise noted, spend at least a minute with each exercise, doing about 10 slow repetitions of each. When completing repetitions, listen to your body. Go slowly, move fluidly, and stop when you've had enough.

These exercises will stretch and strengthen the muscles needed for you to advance to the Complete Pilates Program or to my 3-Week Total Body Makeover in part 4. Stick with the beginner program for about 3 weeks, or as long as it takes for you to feel comfortable doing the exercises. Generally, most people find they can adopt a new habit in 3 weeks, so make that your goal. You can do it!

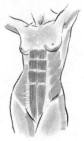

Warmup Stretch with Knee Sway

Benefits

This warms up your back and abs, particularly your outer abs, for the rest of this Pilates routine. In other routines, it also serves as a great stretch for relaxing between tough Pilates movements.

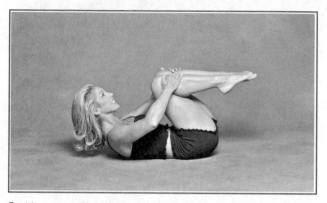

A. Lie on your back with your knees pulled in toward your chest. Hold your shins with your hands. Press your abs toward your spine and allow your lower back to lengthen and widen. Hold the stretch as you inhale and exhale three deep, slow breaths.

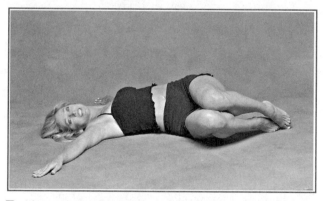

B. Move your hands away from your legs and place them on the floor at shoulder level. Using your abdominal muscles to initiate the move, slowly lower your legs and then bring your knees to the right, as shown, pressing your knees together as you move. Relax and allow your lower back to stretch as you keep your abs pressed toward your spine. Hold the stretch as you inhale and exhale three deep, slow breaths.

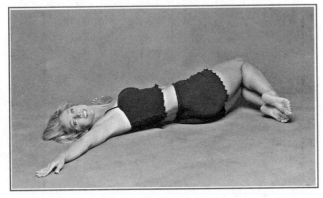

C. Use your abs to pull your knees back to center and then to lower them to the left. Hold the stretch as you inhale and exhale three deep, slow breaths.

Pilates Pointers

► Keep your knees together throughout the move.

► This move should feel good in your lower back. If it doesn't, you're not initiating the movement with your belly.

Denise-eology . . .

"Never underestimate your power to change and improve. You are a good person, with wonderful qualities, and you *can* reach your goals."

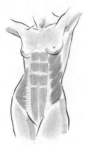

Basic Ab Strengthener

Benefits

This will help increase circulation as well as strengthen your abs, particularly your upper abs, for tougher Pilates moves.

Pilates Pointers

► Resist the tendency to work your upper body in this exercise. Relax your arms, and don't use them to pull your head and shoulders up. If your shoulders rise less than an inch, that's okay. Just do your best.

► Your entire focus during this exercise should be on your abdominals.

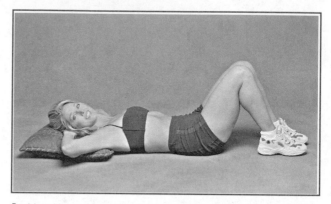

A. Lie with your back on the floor and your head and neck supported by a pillow or cushion. Your knees should be bent with your feet flat on the floor. Place your hands behind your head with your elbows out to the sides.

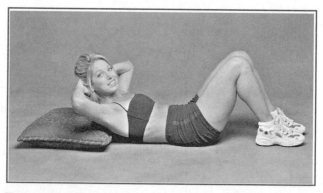

B. Press your abs down to your spine and exhale as you curl your ribs toward your hipbones. Inhale as you lower to the floor. Keep your navel flat throughout the exercise. Repeat.

Lower Ab Strengthener

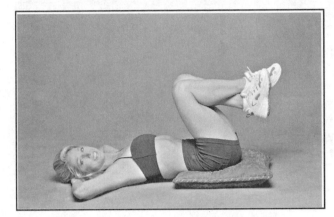

A. Lie with your back on the floor and position a pillow or cushion under your hips and buttocks for added support. Raise your legs and bend your knees, crossing your legs at the ankles. Place your hands behind your head. Your elbows should be out to the sides.

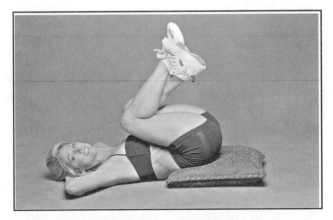

B. Press your abs toward your spine and exhale as you curl your hipbones toward your ribs, initiating the movement with your lower abs. Inhale as you lower your hips. Repeat.

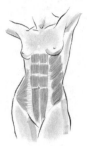

Benefit

This prepares your lower abs—the lower end of your rectus abdominis, a traditional weak spot in women particularly after pregnancy—for tougher Pilates work that follows.

Pilates Pointers

► You should feel this mostly in your lower abs and groin, not your ribs and upper abs.

► Before lifting your hips, tighten and pull the muscles in your groin up, as if you were holding a penny between your legs in your groin area. Then press your navel down. Doing just those two movements will strengthen your abs, even if your hips don't noticeably rise.

► Relax your head into your fingertips and keep your elbows out of sight.

Lower Ab Strengthener

More challenging

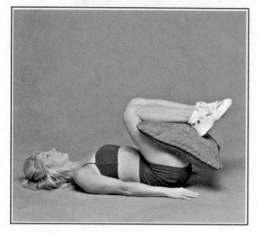

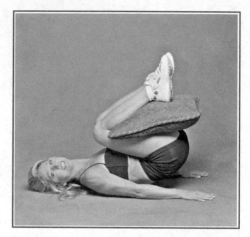

A. If you can do the first variation easily, try this. Lie with your back on the floor, your hands down at your sides, and a pillow or cushion held between your thighs and calves. Lengthen your body from the crown of your head to your tailbone.

B. Press your abs toward your spine and exhale as you curl your hipbones toward your ribs. Inhale as you lower your hips. Repeat.

Denise-eology . . .

"Maintain focus below the belly button. You only need to make a small motion to achieve a maximum effect."

Comfort Ab Curl

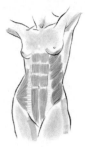

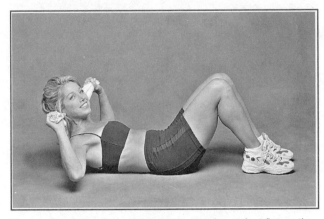

Lie on your back with your knees bent and your feet flat on the floor. Place a rolled-up towel under the base of your head. Grab the ends of the towel. Flatten your abs toward your spine and exhale as you curl up, as shown. If your neck strains, relax it back into the towel. Roll back down to the floor as you inhale. Repeat.

Benefits

Many of the Pilates exercises in the Complete Pilates Program require you to use your abdominals without supporting your neck. So you need strong neck muscles before moving on to that program. If you feel your neck straining when you do Pilates, use a towel, as suggested in this exercise. The towel especially helps those with tight or weak neck muscles, often due to an injury.

Pilates Pointers

► You can use the towel for most Pilates moves. Try to wean yourself off it by holding your head up without the towel and then relaxing it back when your neck becomes tired.

► Remember, faster is not better! Moving slower incorporates more muscle fibers.

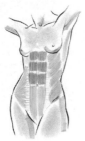

One-Leg Lift

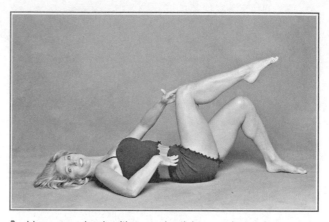

A. Lie on your back with your abs tight, your knees bent, and your feet flat on the floor. Exhale as you lift your right knee up while keeping your hips motionless and level. Use your right hand to make sure your right hip stays in place. Inhale and reach toward your right knee with your left hand, as shown.

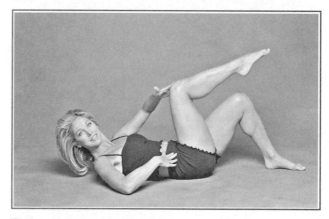

B. Exhale as you use your abs to pull your shoulders up, as shown. Keep your head aligned with your shoulders. Don't lead with your chin. Inhale and lower your shoulders to the floor. Repeat the sequence, switching arm and leg positions. Continue to alternate legs and arms, doing 10 repetitions with each leg using perfect form.

Benefits

This beginner pose will help you build lower abdominal strength as well as help you learn the basic Pilates abdominal posture. It's great for the sides of your waistline, your obliques.

Pilates Pointers

► Keep your hips level and motionless throughout the move.

► If your neck strains during this move, relax the back of your head against your right fingertips. But don't use your fingertips to pull your head forward.

► Keep your abs strong and still. The only parts of your body that should move are your arms and legs.

Sliding Leg

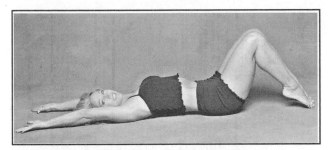

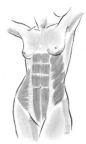

Lie on your back with your arms extended overhead, palms up, and with your knees bent, as shown. Exhale as you slide your pointed right foot out along the floor, only as far as you can keep your abs contracted, making certain that your lower back is flat and pressed into the mat. Bring your knee back in toward your chest as you inhale. Repeat three times and then switch legs.

More challenging

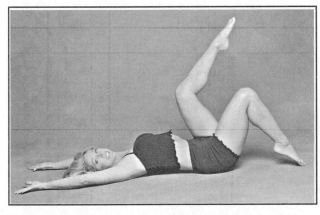

Lie on your back with your arms extended overhead, palms up, and with your knees bent. Point your toes. Bring your left knee in toward your chest, as shown. Exhale as you slowly slide your pointed right foot out along the floor as you keep your abs tight. Slide no farther than you can with your abs contracted, making certain that your lower back is flat and pressed into the mat. Now, bring your right leg in toward your chest as you inhale and slide your left leg out. Continue to alternate your legs, repeating the entire sequence three times.

Benefits

This pose will help you learn how to keep your abs strong and contracted even when your body is lengthening. This will also warm up your hip flexors, in your pelvis, for subsequent movements as well as prepare you to progress to the single-leg stretch (page 51) and other Pilates moves.

Pilates Pointers

► Concentrate on your abs throughout this move. Eventually, you want to fully extend your legs, but with your abs still engaged.

► Keep your abs still. You're only moving your legs.

► Only go as far as the strength in your abs allows.

► Relax your head, neck, and buttocks throughout the move.

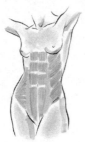

Beginner Hundred

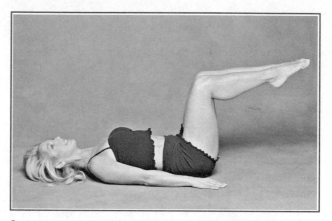

A. Lie with your back on the floor, your arms down at your sides, and your knees in the air, directly above your hips. Extend your calves so that they are parallel to the floor.

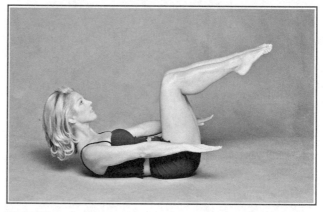

B. Exhale as you contract your abs to lift your shoulders. Inhale. Press your palms down rhythmically as you exhale 5 short breaths, pressing your palms slightly down with each breath. Then turn your palms up and press up rhythmically with 5 short inhales to complete one set. Repeat the sequence as many as 10 times, equaling 100 breaths in all. (If you're just starting out, aim for 20 breaths and eventually increase to 100.)

Benefits

This breathing exercise strengthens the abdominal region as well as warms you up for your Pilates routine.

Beginner Hundred

More challenging

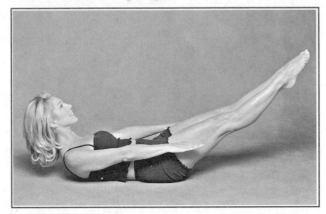

Lie with your back on the floor, your arms down at your sides, and your knees in the air, directly above your hips. Extend your legs and point your toes. Exhale as you contract your abs to pull your shoulders up, as shown. Inhale. Press your palms down rhythmically as you exhale 5 short breaths, pressing your palms slightly down with each breath. Then turn your palms up and press up rhythmically with 5 short inhales to complete one set. Repeat the sequence 10 times, equaling 100 breaths in all.

Even more challenging

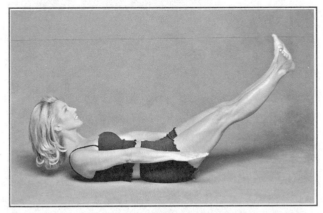

Do everything the same, only flex your feet and turn your toes out. This will target a deeper section of your lower abs below your navel as well as your inner thighs.

Pilates Pointers

► If you're doing the beginner variation on the opposite page, keep your gaze on your knees throughout the move.

► If your abs are not strong enough to do a complete hundred, rest between sets.

► Think "length." Stretch through your fingertips.

► If your neck strains, support your neck and head with a pillow or cushion.

► Press your lower back into the mat and bring your navel down to maintain support for your spine.

► Keep your rib cage in and drawn down toward your hips.

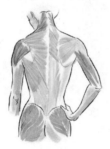

Roll-Ups
Preparation

Benefits

Roll-ups build basic abdominal strength so you can move on to more advanced Pilates exercises. They also stretch the hamstrings (the muscles that form the backs of your thighs) and loosen your spine for subsequent movements. This move improves abdominal control through imprinting. That means you're slowly rolling up one vertebra at a time. Then when you roll down, you're imprinting your spine one vertebra at a time into the mat.

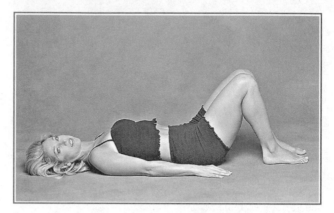

A. Lie on your back with your knees bent and feet flat on the floor. Extend your arms so that your hands rest on either side of your buttocks.

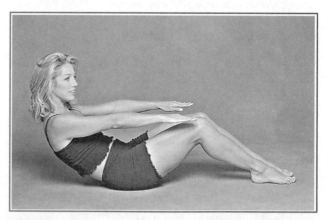

B. Exhale as you contract your tummy and squeeze your inner thighs together to lift your shoulders up, bringing your ribs closer to your hips. Stop once your shoulder blades lift from the floor. Inhale as you release your shoulders to the floor. Repeat three times.

Roll-Ups
Preparation

More challenging

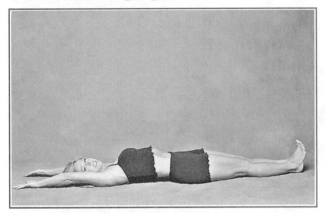

A. Lie on your back with your arms stretched over your head and with your legs extended, feet flexed. Inhale.

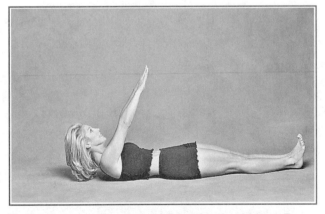

B. Exhale as you bring your arms in front of your chest. Engage your abs and squeeze your inner thighs together to lift your shoulders up, as shown, bringing your ribs closer to your hips. As you roll up, let the movement come from your abs, not from momentum.

Pilates Pointers

► At first, you can use your hands under your bent knees to help yourself rise. Move on to the more challenging version when you no longer need your hands for help.

► Relax your neck and shoulders, and if you're doing the less challenging exercise, on the opposite page, focus your eyes on your knees.

► Imagine yourself scooping out your abdominal area into a C shape.

► This isn't a contest to see how high you can lift your shoulders. Focus on your abs. Lift only as high as your abs can hold out.

► Keep your heels on the floor at all times.

—continued

Roll-Ups Preparation

More challenging—continued

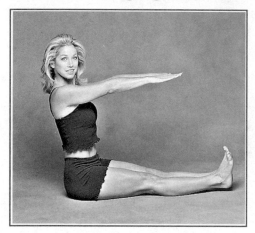

C. Sit tall; check that your abs are pulled in toward your spine as you inhale.

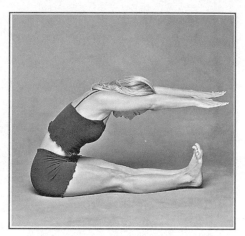

D. Exhale and bend forward, keeping your abs scooped in—that is, pull your navel in toward your spine. Roll back to the starting position, using your abs throughout the movement, and try to feel every single vertebra touch the floor one at a time. Complete three full roll-ups.

Denise-eology . . .

"Imagine you're sitting on a beach,
and as you roll down,
one vertebra at a time,
the bones in your spine make small
indentations in the sand—
that's what we call 'imprinting' in Pilates."

Beginner
Single-Leg Circles

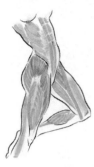

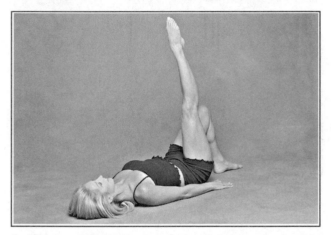

A. Lie on your back with your arms at your sides, your knees bent, and your feet flat on the floor. Extend your right leg and point your toes, as shown. Exhale and tighten your abs, navel in. Press your spine down into the mat.

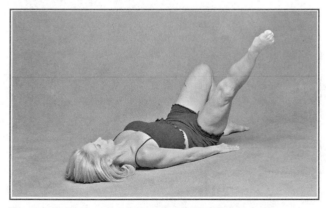

B. Slowly circle your right leg counterclockwise, as shown, making sure to keep your hips level and motionless. Inhale as you circle your leg outward, away from your body. Exhale as you circle inward, toward your body. After circling six times in that direction, switch to clockwise for six circles. Repeat the sequence with the other leg.

Benefits

Leg circles strengthen your inner and outer thighs as well as teach you how to stabilize your abs and hips during circular movements.

Pilates Pointers

► Keep both buttocks on the floor at all times.

► Keep your abs completely still.

► Imagine that you are drawing a circle on the ceiling with your big toe.

► Draw small circles at first, then progress to larger circles to help improve flexibility of the muscles surrounding your hip joint.

► Feel as though your hips are anchored to the floor.

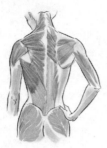

Rolling like a Ball

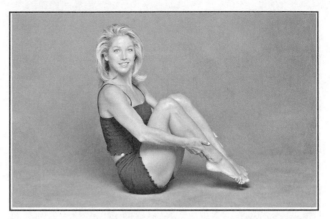

Benefits

This move will help you stretch your spine while teaching you to keep the deepest layer of your abs contracted during movement. It will also improve your balance and massage your spine.

A. Sit with your back flat, abs tight, knees bent, and feet pulled close to your buttocks. Place your hands near your ankles and balance on your "sit bones," as shown, with your feet an inch off the floor. Pull your abs toward your spine to help keep your balance.

Pilates Pointers

► Your body will try to unravel during this move. Focus on keeping your abs pressed against your spine.

► Slow down the move to stay in control. Don't let momentum carry you back and forward. Instead, focus on moving from your abs.

► As you gain more control during this exercise, try to keep your heels close to your buttocks throughout the move.

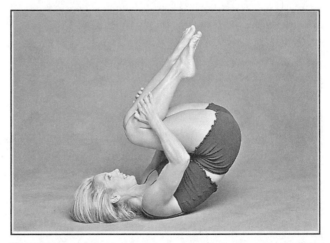

B. While keeping your abs pressed against your spine, inhale as you roll back smoothly until your shoulder blades touch the floor. Then exhale as you roll forward to the starting position. Try not to let your feet touch the floor. Instead, roll into the balanced position on your sit bones. If you're just starting out, allow your toes to slightly touch the floor until you gain more control. Repeat the sequence three to five more times.

Single-Leg Stretch with Pillow

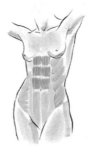

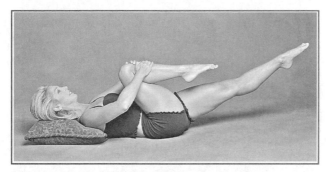

A. Lie on your back with your head and neck resting on a pillow or cushion and your legs extended. Scoop your stomach toward your spine, exhale, and raise your left leg off the floor only as high as you can keep your lower back flat against the floor. Simultaneously, bring your right knee in toward your chest, as shown. Place your right hand on your right knee and your left hand on your right ankle.

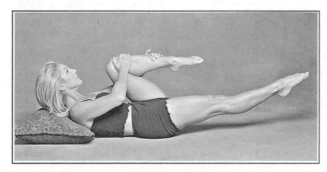

B. Contract your abs and raise your shoulders. Stay in position as you bring your left knee in toward your chest and extend your right leg, as shown. Continue to alternate your arms and legs in the raised position, inhaling as you change legs, exhaling as your knee comes to your chest. Repeat the entire sequence four more times. Relax your shoulders and lower them back to the floor. If you can't keep your shoulders up throughout the move, do some repetitions with your shoulders raised and some with them lowered to the floor.

Benefits

This move will help you learn to stabilize your hips and abs, even when your legs aren't together. It will also boost your coordination and stretch your back and legs.

Pilates Pointers

► Think "length." Extend your straight leg as much as possible. Imagine that a string is pulling your extended big toe away from your body, creating length.

► Press through your inner thighs, as if your thighs were squeezing a cushion.

► Relax your shoulders by pressing your elbows toward your hips.

► Keep your neck open and long, not scrunched toward your chest.

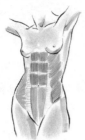

Leg Lift with Reach

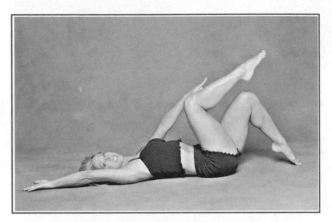

Benefits

This targets your lower abdominals and obliques, the abdominal muscles that form your waist. This exercise prepares you for the next level—the crisscross in the Complete Pilates Program. It's also a great rotation exercise for the waistline.

A. Lie on your back with both knees bent and your arms overhead. Press your abs toward your spine as you raise your right knee toward your chest and your left foot just an inch from the floor. At the same time, raise your left arm toward your right knee, as shown. Inhale and exhale as you switch your arm and leg positions, moving with your breath. Keep your abs engaged throughout the exercise. Continue to alternate your arms and legs, repeating the entire sequence 10 times.

Denise-eology . . .
"Don't forget to keep your abs hunkered down, in an abdominal compression!"

Leg Lift with Reach

More challenging

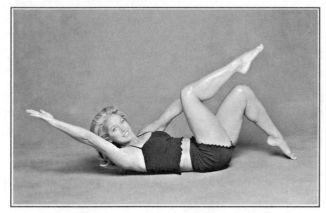

A. From the same starting position, contract your abs and press your ribs toward your hips to raise your shoulders off the floor. Twist your torso slightly to target your oblique muscles.

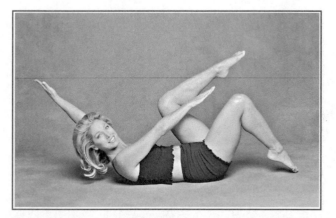

B. Inhale and exhale as you switch your arm and leg positions. Continue to alternate your arms and legs, repeating the entire sequence 10 times.

Pilates Pointers

► Keep your abs pressed toward your spine throughout the move.

► Lengthen through your fingertips as you reach, extending your hands away from each other.

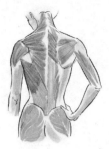

Spine Stretch Forward

Benefits

This exercise is a wonderful stretch for the entire back. Plus, it strengthens your deep abdominals, helping you to sit with good posture. This spine stretch creates space for each vertebra and lengthens the spine. It's also a great stretch for the hamstrings.

Pilates Pointers

► Move first from your abs, bringing them toward your spine and then curling forward from your belly, then ribs, then chest, then neck. Don't lead with your head.

► Many people tense their shoulders during this exercise. Concentrate on keeping your shoulders low, away from your ears.

► Keep your sit bones glued to the floor.

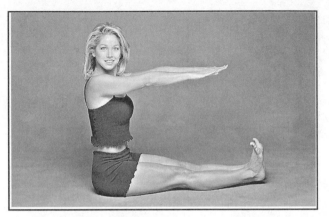

A. Sit with your legs slightly apart and extended in front of you, your feet flexed, and your knees slightly bent. Pull your abs in toward your spine. Extend your arms at chest level, making sure to keep your shoulders relaxed, not hunched over.

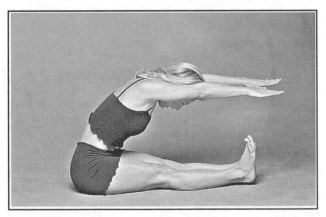

B. Exhale as you bend forward, pulling your abs back against the spine, scooping them into a C shape. Inhale as you roll back to the start, using your abs to pull yourself up. Repeat three times, progressively increasing your flexibility.

Bridge with Pillow

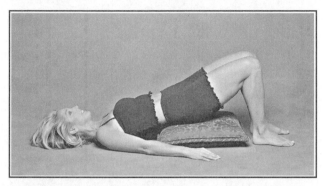

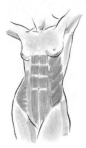

Lie on your back with your knees bent and your feet flat on the floor. Rest your arms at your sides, with your palms down and at about hip level. Place a pillow or cushion under your buttocks for support. Take a deep breath. Exhale as you contract your abs and curl your hips up, as shown, using your abs (not your buttocks or lower back) to lift your torso. You can use your hands for balance, but don't use them to push yourself up. Hold for 10 to 15 seconds, relax, and repeat one time.

More challenging

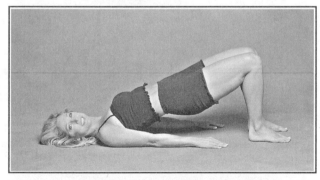

Lie on your back with your knees bent and your feet flat on the floor. Rest your arms at your sides, with your palms down and at about hip level. Take a deep breath. Exhale as you contract your abs and curl your hips up, as shown, using your abs (not your buttocks or lower back) to lift your torso. You can use your hands for balance, but don't use them to push yourself up. Hold for 10 to 15 seconds, relax, and repeat one time.

Benefits

This move teaches you to use your deepest abs, your transverse abdominis, to protect your back when it's in an arched position. It also stretches the hip flexors and strengthens your hamstrings, firming the backs of your thighs and buttocks.

Pilates Pointers

► Imagine curling your hip-bones toward your ribs. This will prevent you from arching your back too much. Your abs should appear scooped in, not pushed out.

► Contract your abs, starting at your groin, all the way up to your ribs. But keep your buttocks and lower back relaxed.

► When in the raised position, lengthen your torso by extending your hips toward your feet.

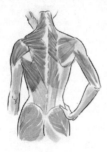

Back Reliever with Pillow

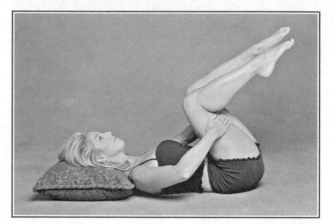

Lie on your back with your head and neck supported by a pillow or cushion and your knees bent and feet on the floor. Use the strength of your abs to pull your thighs in toward your chest. Wrap your arms around the backs of your thighs, as shown, pulling your legs closer to your chest. Take a deep breath and then exhale with a sigh. Hold the stretch for 15 seconds, relax, and repeat one time.

Benefits

For optimum balance, this move provides the opposite movement of the bridge (page 55) to let your spine relax and lengthen. This feels wonderful.

Pilates Pointer

► Press your abs toward your spine to fully open your lower back.

Denise-eology . . .

"If your abs are strong, chances are the rest of your body is totally fit."

Abdominal Lengthener

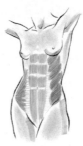

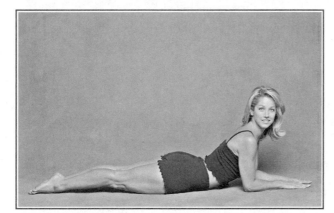

Lie on your tummy with your legs extended, your hands beside your shoulders, and your upper arms close to your body. Scoop your abs toward your back so that your pubic bone presses into the floor but your abs scoop away from the floor. With your abs in position, raise your chest and shoulders off the floor, as shown, pulling slightly forward with your palms to keep your chest open and your shoulders low. Inhale and exhale as you hold the stretch for 15 seconds. Relax and repeat one time.

Benefits

This move strengthens and stretches your abs as well as lengthens your lower spine. It also prepares and stretches your belly for the next move, the back strengthener.

Pilates Pointers

► Keep your shoulders relaxed, away from your ears.

► Keep your abs scooped in toward your spine throughout the move.

► Your buttocks should remain relatively relaxed in this pose, with only a slight contraction near your groin.

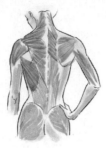

Benefits

Great for your back muscles that line your spine, this move teaches you to keep your abs pressed toward your spine as you extend through your back.

Pilates Pointers

► Press your fingertips forward and your toes back to create more length in your spine. Think "long," not "high."

► Press your abs in toward your spine to prevent your lower back from arching.

► Keep your abs engaged. Don't let your tummy hang down—pull it up and in.

Back Strengthener

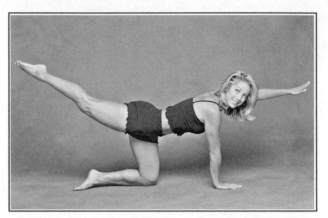

Get on all fours, with your hands under your shoulders and your knees under your hips. Press your navel toward your spine and lengthen the crown of your head toward the wall in front of you and your tailbone toward the wall behind you. Inhale as you extend your left arm and right leg, as shown. Hold for 2 seconds, then exhale as you lower. Repeat using your right arm and left leg. Continue alternating arm and leg positions, repeating the entire sequence two more times.

Denise-eology . . .
"If you start moving your body, your mind will follow."

Total Rest Pose

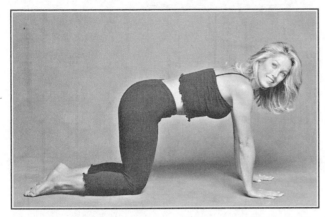

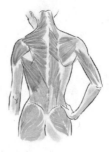

A. Get on your hands and knees, with your abs tight and your back flat. Your hands should be directly under your shoulders and your knees directly under your hips, with the tops of your feet flat on the floor.

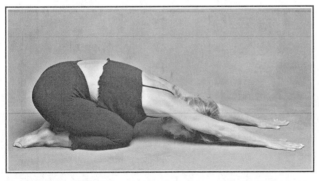

B. From your belly move back, bringing your buttocks onto the tops of your heels and resting your belly on your thighs. Keep your hands rooted in position throughout the move. Inhale and exhale as you relax, holding the pose for 30 seconds.

Benefits

The total rest pose does just that—it relaxes your back. In this pose, your spine is long. It's a great pose to do as a warmup or simply a rest between tough Pilates poses.

Pilates Pointers

► Keep your shoulder blades spread apart from one another. It should feel as if your thumbs and index fingers want to lift up from the floor, but keep them pressed down.

► When bringing your hips back, pull in your belly button toward your spine. This action will allow you to further extend your buttocks to your heels.

► Breathe into your ribs, using your breath to expand your back, not your lower belly or chest.

THE Beginner Pilates PROGRAM at a Glance

Complete the beginner program in sequence three times a week until you feel balanced, strong, and flexible when doing the moves. From there, you can move on to the Complete Pilates Program, in the next chapter. Or you can tackle the exercises in the 3-Week Total Body Makeover in part 4. Try to flow from exercise to exercise, moving with your breath.

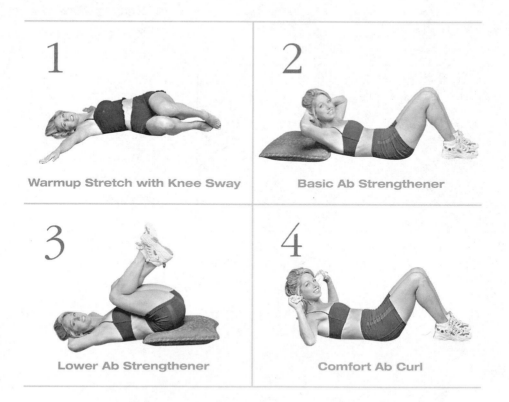

1 Warmup Stretch with Knee Sway

2 Basic Ab Strengthener

3 Lower Ab Strengthener

4 Comfort Ab Curl

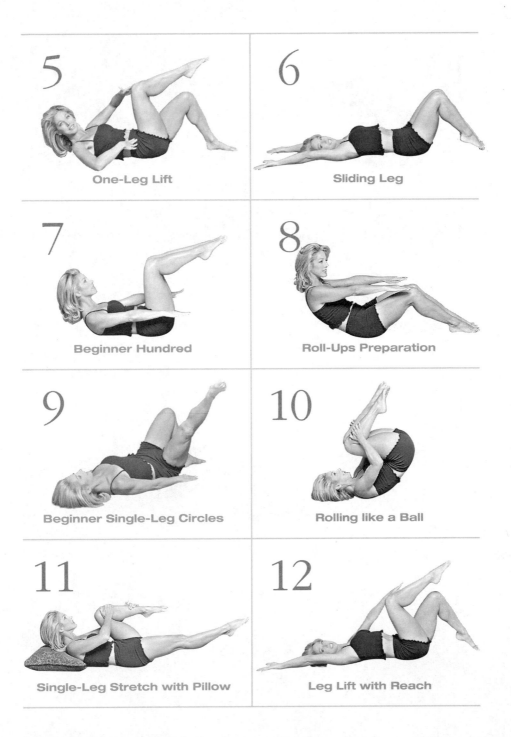

5 One-Leg Lift

6 Sliding Leg

7 Beginner Hundred

8 Roll-Ups Preparation

9 Beginner Single-Leg Circles

10 Rolling like a Ball

11 Single-Leg Stretch with Pillow

12 Leg Lift with Reach

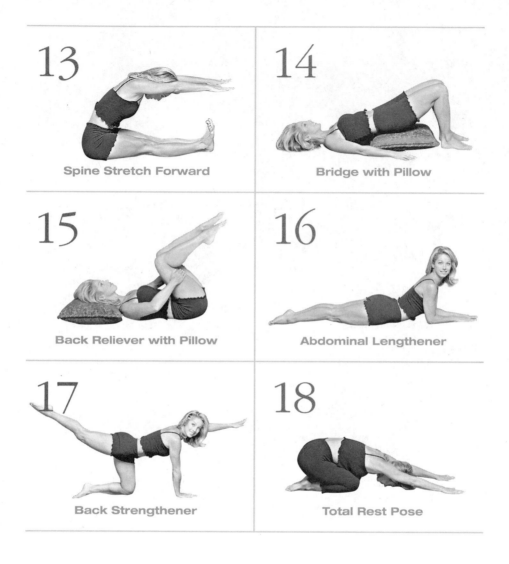

13 Spine Stretch Forward

14 Bridge with Pillow

15 Back Reliever with Pillow

16 Abdominal Lengthener

17 Back Strengthener

18 Total Rest Pose

The COMPLETE Pilates PROGRAM

This routine provides you with a sequence of movements that flow from one exercise to the next. You should feel smooth and fluid during your transition between moves. If you feel awkward in some of these exercises at first, know that in time your strength, flexibility, coordination, breathing, and balance will come together, helping you to mindfully move from pose to pose.

Completing all of these movements in order can be challenging, even for me. Try the Complete Pilates Program after you've already mastered the Beginner Pilates Program on page 35. As in the Beginner Pilates Program, some exercises have two or more versions. If you're just moving from the beginner program, start with the less challenging versions then work your way up to the more challenging.

Unless otherwise noted, try to spend at least a minute with every move, doing about 10 slow repetitions. Listen to your body when completing repetitions. Go slowly, move fluidly, and give 110 percent of effort. Think "quality" over "quantity."

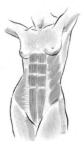

Warmup Stretch with Knee Sway

Benefits

This warms up your back and abs, particularly your outer abs, for the rest of your Pilates routine. The warmup stretch is a great stretch for relaxing between tough Pilates movements.

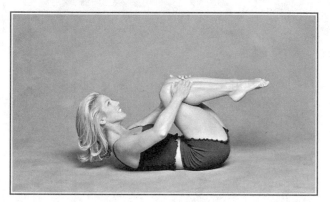

A. Lie on your back with your knees pulled in toward your chest. Hold your shins with your hands. Press your abs toward your spine and allow your lower back to lengthen and widen. Hold the stretch as you inhale and exhale three deep, slow breaths.

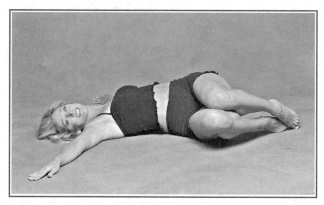

B. Move your hands away from your legs and place them on the floor at shoulder level. Using your abdominal muscles to initiate the move, slowly lower your legs and then bring your knees to the right, as shown, pressing your knees together as you move. Relax and allow your lower back to stretch as you keep your abs pressed toward your spine. Hold the stretch as you inhale and exhale three deep, slow breaths.

► Keep your knees together throughout the move.

► This move should feel good in your lower back. If it doesn't, you're not initiating the movement with your belly.

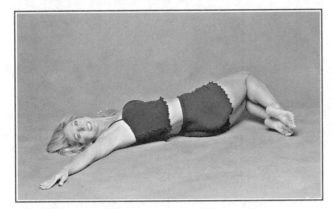

C. Use your abs to pull your knees back to center and then to lower them to the left. Hold the stretch as you inhale and exhale three deep, slow breaths.

Denise-eology . . .

"When you approach Pilates with confidence, you will perform beyond your expectations."

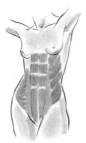

The Hundred

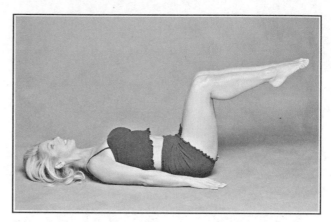

A. Lie with your back on the floor, your arms down at your sides, and your knees in the air, directly above your hips. Extend your calves so that they are parallel to the floor.

Benefits

This breathing exercise strengthens your abs as well as warms you up for your Pilates routine.

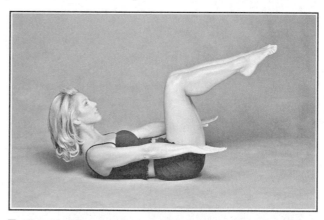

B. Exhale as you contract your abs to lift your shoulders. Inhale. Press your palms down rhythmically as you exhale 5 short breaths, pressing your palms slightly down with each breath. Then turn your palms up and press up rhythmically with 5 short inhales to complete one set. Repeat the sequence as many as 10 times, equaling 100 breaths in all. (If you're just starting out, aim for 20 breaths and eventually increase to 100.)

The Hundred

More challenging

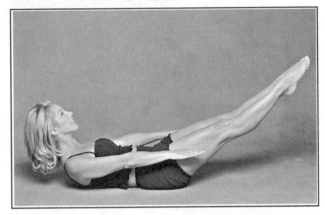

Lie with your back on the floor, your arms down at your sides, and your knees in the air, directly above your hips. Extend your legs and point your toes. Exhale as you contract your abs to pull your shoulders up, as shown. Inhale. Press your palms down rhythmically as you exhale 5 short breaths, pressing your palms slightly down with each breath. Then turn your palms up and press up rhythmically with 5 short inhales to complete one set. Repeat the sequence 10 times, equaling 100 breaths in all.

Even more challenging

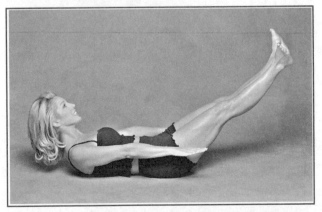

Do everything the same, only flex your feet and turn your toes out. This will target a deeper section of your lower abs below your navel and tone your inner thighs.

Pilates Pointers

► If you're doing the beginner variation, on the opposite page, keep your gaze on your knees throughout the move.

► If your abs lack the strength to do a complete hundred, rest between sets.

► Think "length." Stretch through your fingertips.

► If your neck strains, support your neck and head with a pillow or cushion.

► Press your lower back into the mat and bring your navel down to maintain support for your spine.

► Keep your rib cage in and drawn down toward your hips.

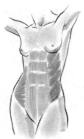

The Roll-Up

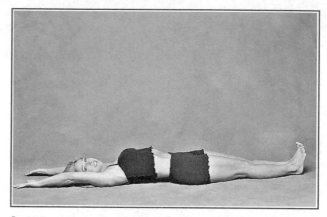

A. Lie on your back with your arms stretched over your head and with your legs extended, feet flexed. Inhale.

Benefits

A great exercise for your hard-to-target transverse abdominis around your belt, the roll-up builds basic abdominal strength so you can move on to more advanced exercises. It also stretches the hamstrings (the muscles that form the backs of your thighs) and the individual vertebra in your spine, readying them for subsequent movements.

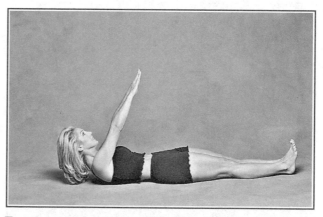

B. Exhale as you bring your arms in front of your chest. Engage your abs and squeeze your inner thighs together to lift your shoulders up, as shown, bringing your ribs closer to your hips. As you roll up, let the movement come from your abs, not from momentum. Keep your chin to your chest as you roll up to a sitting position.

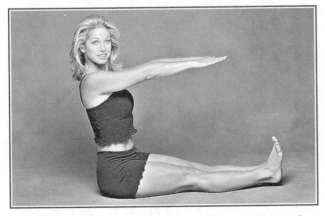

C. Sit tall; check that your abs are pulled in toward your spine as you inhale.

Pilates Pointers

► Relax your neck and shoulders.

► Imagine yourself scooping out your abdominal area into a C shape.

► Keep your heels on the floor at all times.

► Feel yourself "imprinting" as you roll down one vertebra at a time. And as you roll up, feel yourself "peeling" back up.

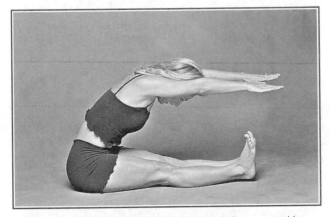

D. Exhale and bend forward, keeping your abs scooped in— that is, pull your navel in toward your spine. Roll back to the starting position, using your abs throughout the movement, and try to feel every single vertebra touch the floor one at a time. Complete three full roll-ups.

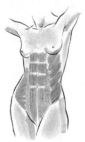

Bridge

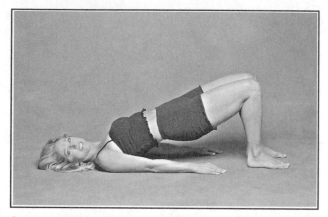

A. Lie on your back with your knees bent and your feet flat on the floor. Rest your arms at your sides, with your palms down and at about hip level. Take a deep breath. Exhale as you contract your abs and curl your hips up, as shown, using your abs (not your buttocks or lower back) to lift your torso. You can use your hands for balance, but don't use them to push yourself up.

Benefits

This move teaches you to use your abs to protect your back when it's in an arched position. It also stretches the hip flexors in your pelvis and strengthens the hamstrings.

Denise-eology . . .

"This will help reshape your bottom half to make it your best half."

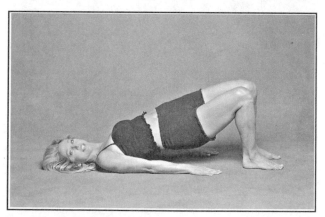

B. From the bridge position, move your hips slightly toward the right. If you keep your abs scooped, you should feel this in your lower left abdominal area. Repeat on the other side, then repeat the entire sequence one time.

Bridge

More challenging

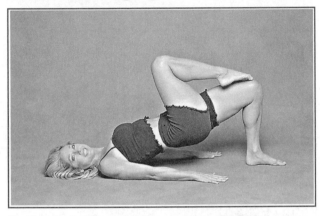

A. From the bridge position, press your navel toward your spine as you lift your right knee toward your belly.

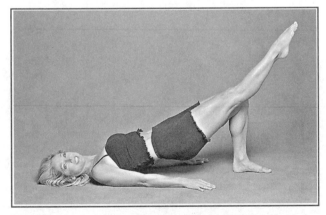

B. With your navel still pressed toward your spine, extend your leg through your right toes, keeping your body in a straight line. Relax and repeat with the other leg, then repeat the sequence one time.

Pilates Pointers

► Imagine curling your hip-bones toward your ribs. This will prevent you from arching your back too much. Your abs should appear scooped in, not pushed out.

► Contract your abs, starting at your groin, all the way up to your ribs. But keep your buttocks and lower back relaxed.

► When in the raised position, lengthen your torso by extending your hips toward your feet.

► Keep your abs engaged.

Single-Leg Circles

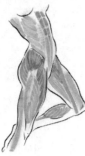

Benefits

Leg circles trim and tone your inner and outer thighs as well as teach you how to stabilize your abs and hips during circular movements. They also prepare your lower abs for subsequent movements in this program.

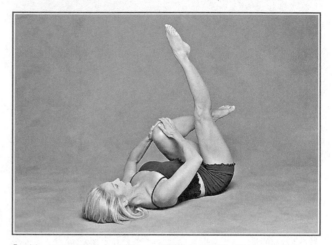

A. Lie on your back, with your left knee pulled in toward your chest, both hands resting just below the knee, and your right leg extended, toes pointed.

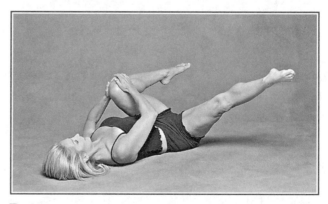

B. Circle your right leg counterclockwise, as shown, making sure to keep your hips level and motionless. Inhale as you circle your leg outward, away from your body. Exhale as you circle it toward your body. Once you've made three complete revolutions, switch direction, circling clockwise three times. Then switch legs and repeat the sequence.

Single-Leg Circles

More challenging

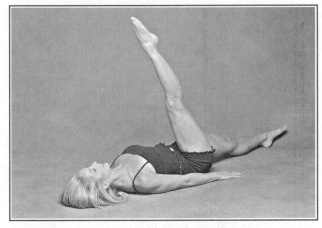

A. Lie on your back with your arms down at your sides and with both legs extended, toes pointed. Lift your right leg and extend through your abs.

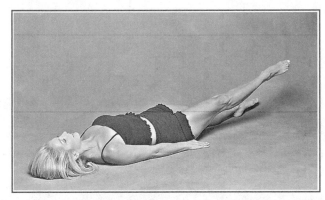

B. Circle your right leg counterclockwise, making sure to keep your hips level and motionless. Inhale as you circle your leg away from your body. Exhale as you circle it toward your body. Once you've made three complete revolutions, reverse direction, circling clockwise three times. Then switch legs and repeat the sequence.

Pilates Pointers

► Keep both buttocks on the floor at all times.

► Keep your abs completely still and anchor your hips to the floor.

► Imagine that you are drawing a circle on the ceiling with your big toe.

► Draw small circles at first, advancing to larger circles as you gain control over your hips.

Denise-eology . . .

"Think about lengthening your legs. Imagine them longer as you reach through your toes."

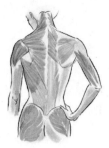

Rolling like a Ball

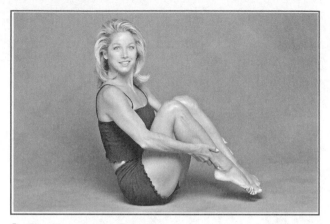

Benefits

This move will help you stretch your spine while teaching you to keep your deepest abs contracted during movement. It will also improve your balance and massage your spine.

Pilates Pointers

► Your body will try to unravel during this move. Focus on keeping your abs pressed against your spine.

► Slow down the move to stay in control. Don't let momentum carry you back and forward. Instead, focus on moving from your abs.

► As you gain more control of the rolling momentum, try to keep your heels close to your buttocks throughout the move.

A. Sit with your back flat, abs tight, knees bent, and feet pulled close to your buttocks. Place your hands near your ankles and balance on your "sit bones," as shown, with your feet an inch off the floor. Pull your abs toward your spine to help keep your balance.

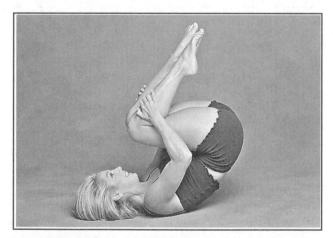

B. While keeping your abs pressed against your spine, inhale as you roll back smoothly until your shoulder blades touch the floor. Then exhale as you roll forward to the starting position. Don't allow your feet to touch the floor. Instead, roll back to the balanced position on your sit bones. Repeat three to five more times.

Single-Leg Stretch

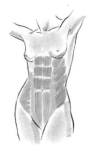

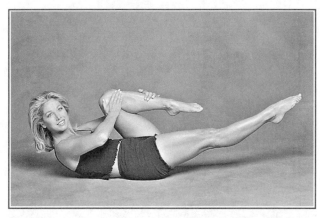

A. Lie on your back with your legs extended. With your abs tight, exhale and raise your right leg off the floor only as high as you can keep your lower back flat against the floor. At the same time, bring your left knee in toward your chest. Place your right hand on your left knee and your left hand on your left ankle, as shown. Contract your abs and raise your shoulders.

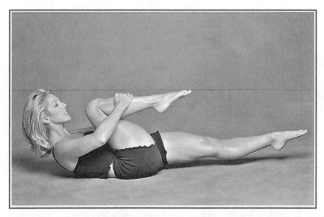

B. Without lowering your head to the floor, bring your right knee in toward your chest and extend your left leg. Continue to alternate your arms and legs in the raised position, inhaling as you change legs and exhaling as your knee comes to your chest. Repeat the entire sequence five to eight times. Relax your shoulders and lower them back to the floor.

Benefits

Great for your entire abdominal area, this move will help you learn to stabilize your hips and abs, even when your legs aren't together. It will also boost your coordination and stretch your back and legs, preparing you perfectly for the very next move, the double-leg stretch.

Pilates Pointers

► Think "length." Extend your straight leg as much as possible. Imagine that a string is pulling your big toe away from your body.

► Press through your inner thighs, as if your thighs were squeezing a cushion.

► Relax your shoulders by pressing your elbows toward your hips.

► Keep your neck open and long, not scrunched toward your chest.

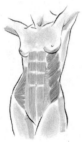

Double-Leg Stretch

Benefits

A fantastic ab strengthener, this move will teach you how to keep your abs contracted as your body's center of gravity moves. It will also teach you to coordinate your breathing with arm and leg movements. As a bonus, it stretches your arms and legs.

Pilates Pointers

► This move will test your lower abdominal strength. It's better to not fully extend your arms and legs—to help keep your abs tight and back flat—than it is to fully extend but arch your back.

► Imagine that your pubic bone and rib cage are moving away from each other and that a heavy brick is keeping you from rounding your tummy.

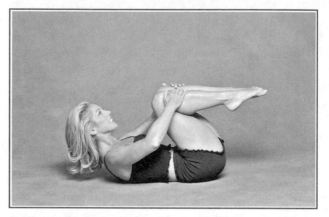

A. Lie on your back with your knees pulled in toward your chest. Rest your hands just below your knees and inhale as you use your abs to raise your shoulders off the floor.

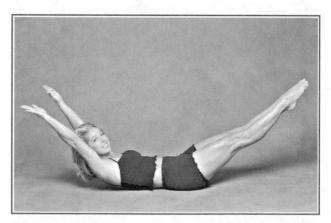

B. Exhale as you press your arms and legs out, making sure to engage and move from your abs. Extend through your finger-tips and toes, as shown. Inhale as you bring your knees back toward your chest and your arms back toward your knees. Repeat five to eight times.

Single Straight-Leg Stretch

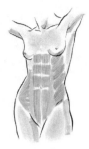

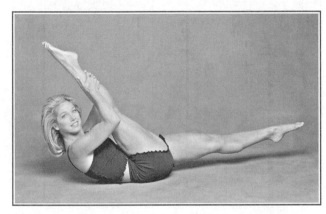

A. Lie on your back with your knees pulled in toward your chest. Pull your abs toward your spine as you exhale and raise your shoulders from the floor. Extend your right leg toward the ceiling and grab your right calf or ankle with both hands. At the same time, extend your left leg in front of you, as shown. Point both feet, drawing both big toes out away from your body.

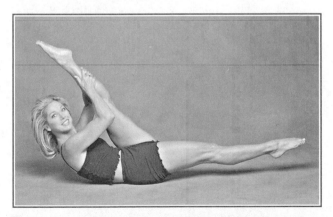

B. Inhale and switch your legs so that your left leg is near your chest and your right leg is extended. Be sure to move as you inhale and exhale. Continue to alternate legs, repeating the entire sequence five to eight times. Try percussion breathing, described on page 33, if needed.

Benefits

The third and more difficult of this progressive series of leg stretches and ab strengtheners, the straight-leg stretch fully lengthens the hamstrings and also targets the entire abdominal region. Great for your legs, too.

Pilates Pointers

► Keep your hips stable throughout the move.

► Keep your navel pulled in toward your spine at all times.

► Keep your shoulders relaxed and your abs engaged.

Denise-eology . . .

"Imagine that your abs are 'zipped in' like a corset."

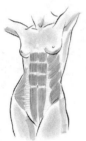

Crisscross

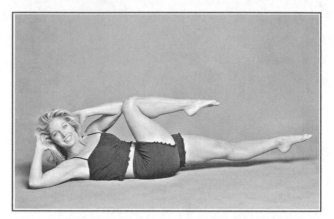

Benefit

This strengthens the obliques, the abdominal muscles that form your waist, preparing them for subsequent twisting movements.

Pilates Pointers

▶ Keep your shoulder blades off the floor throughout the move. Make sure that they are pressed down and back, so your shoulders don't hunch toward your ears.

▶ Press out through the toes of your extended leg, as if someone were pulling your big toe with a string.

▶ You should not be able to see your elbows. If you can, open them more to the side.

▶ Plant your hips down toward the floor to keep them level and motionless.

▶ Keep your torso anchored to the floor.

Lie on your back with your head resting back into your fingertips. Your elbows should be open to the sides. Bend your knees, placing your feet flat on the floor. Contract your abs and lift both feet off the floor. Exhale as you extend your left leg and simultaneously bring your right knee toward your chest. At the same time, rotate your shoulders, bringing your left elbow toward your right knee, as shown. Inhale as you change positions. Once your shoulder almost reaches the floor, exhale and repeat the move by extending your right leg and bringing your left knee in toward your chest. Repeat the entire sequence five to eight times.

Denise-eology . . .

"You should feel this move in your powerhouse— your abs, waistline, and torso— not your neck or shoulders."

Spine Stretch Forward

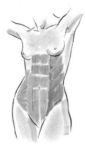

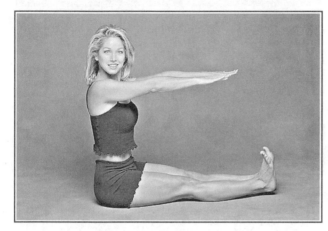

A. Sit with your legs extended in front of you, your feet flexed, and your knees slightly bent. Pull your abs in toward your spine. Extend your arms in front of you at chest level, making sure to keep your shoulders relaxed.

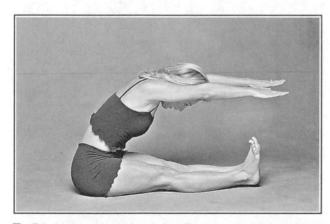

B. Exhale as you bend forward, pulling your abs back against the spine while you bend, scooping your abs into a C shape. Inhale as you roll back to the start, using your abs to pull yourself up. Repeat three times, progressively increasing your flexibility.

Benefit

Strengthens your deep abdominals, your transverse abdominis, helping you to sit with good posture.

Pilates Pointers

► Many people hunch their shoulders during this exercise. Concentrate on keeping them low, away from your ears.

► Move first from your abs, bringing them toward your spine to curl your body forward. Allow your abs to move first, then your ribs, then your chest, then your neck.

Denise-eology . . .

"As you roll back up, scoop in your abs even more, creating more space between each vertebra."

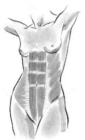

The Saw

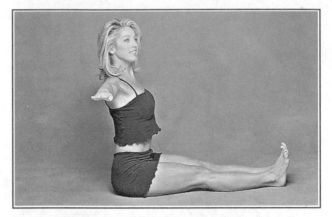

A. Sit with your legs extended hip width apart, feet flexed, and your arms extended out to the sides at chest level. Pull your abs toward your spine and feel yourself sitting on your sit bones.

Benefits

This move stretches the spine as it rotates as well as strengthens the sides of your torso. The breathing technique for the move forces you to push stale air from deep in your lower lungs.

Pilates Pointers

► As you reach forward, rotate from your ribs and turn your chest toward the ceiling.

► Throughout the move, lengthen through the crown of your head, as if someone were pulling it up with a string.

► Keep both hips pressed into the floor. Don't let either buttock rise.

► Scoop in your abs.

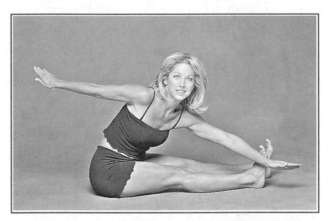

B. Exhale as you reach your left hand toward your right foot, as shown, trying to "saw" off your foot with your pinkie. As you reach for your toe, contract your abs to push all of the air out of your lungs. Inhale as you return to the starting position and repeat on the other side. Continue alternating sides, repeating the sequence two more times.

Abdominal Stretch

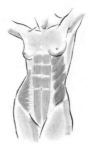

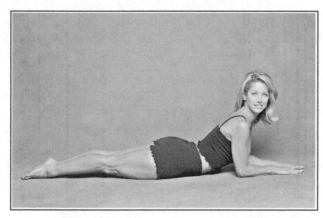

Lie on your belly with your legs extended, your hands beside your shoulders, and your upper arms close to your body. Scoop your abs toward your back so that your pubic bone presses into the floor, but your abs scoop away from the floor. With your abs in position, raise your chest and shoulders off the floor, as shown, pulling slightly forward with your palms to keep your chest open and your shoulders low. Inhale and exhale as you hold for 5 to 10 seconds, then relax and repeat once more.

Benefits

This move strengthens and lengthens your abs as well as increases flexibility through your lower back.

Pilates Pointers

► Keep your shoulders relaxed, away from your ears.

► Keep your abs scooped in toward your spine throughout the move.

► Your buttocks should be lightly tightened, with a slight contraction near your groin.

Denise-eology . . .

"Between abdominal stretch sets,
I like to do a total rest pose (page 59)
to stretch my lower back
in the opposite direction.
It truly feels wonderful."

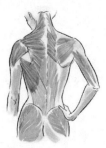

Leg Raise

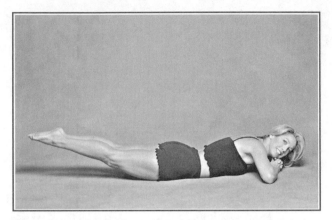

Lie on your tummy, fold your arms in front of you, and rest your head into your folded arms. Scoop your abs up against your spine so that your pubic bone presses into the floor. Lengthen your legs by pressing through your toes as you raise your heels up, as shown. If lifting both legs feels too difficult, try just one leg at a time. Hold for 3 to 5 seconds and remember to breathe. Relax and repeat one time.

Benefits

Leg raises strengthen and stretch your abs, strengthen your lower back, and elongate your lower spine. They prepare you for the next exercise, the Superman.

Pilates Pointers

► If you feel any pinching or strain in your lower back, your abs are not pressed firmly against your spine.

► Keep your buttocks tight, contracting in your groin area, too.

Denise-eology . . .

"Commit yourself to constant self-improvement. The joy is truly in the journey."

Superman

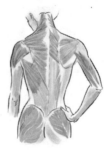

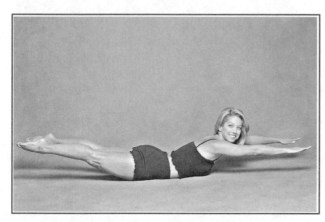

Lie on your belly, with your arms extended in front of you and your legs extended back. Scoop your abs up against your spine so that your pubic bone presses into the floor. Lengthen through your legs and arms by pressing through your toes and fingers as you raise your heels up and shoulders up, as shown. Squeeze your buttocks to prevent your lower back from arching. Hold for 3 to 5 seconds, remembering to breathe and using the "two inhales, two exhales" technique described on page 33. Relax and repeat one time.

Benefits

Strengthens and stretches your abs, strengthens your entire back, and elongates your spine.

Pilates Pointers

► If you feel any pinching or strain in your lower back, your abs are not pressed firmly against your spine.

► Keep your buttocks tight, contracting in your groin area, too.

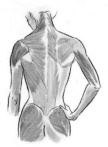

Benefits

This move strengthens and stretches your back besides teaching you to support your back with your abs, even when it's slightly arched.

Pilates Pointers

► Keep your shoulders relaxed, with your shoulder blades pressed down, not hunched up toward your ears.

► Though your back does some work in this move, concentrate on pressing and moving from your abs.

► Keep your buttocks tight, contracting in your groin area, too.

► Press through your fingers and toes to further lengthen your body.

Swimming

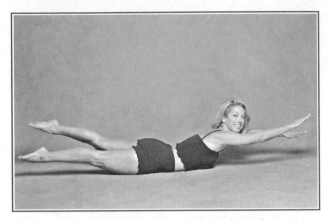

Lie on your belly with your arms extended in front of you and your legs extended back. Press through your fingertips and toes to create length in your spine. Inhale as you raise your right arm and left leg a few inches higher than your left arm and right leg, as shown. Exhale as you switch positions, lowering your right arm and left leg and raising your left arm and right leg. Continue alternating your arms and legs, as if you were swimming, repeating the entire sequence five to nine times.

Denise-eology . . .
"You are creating a body that is strong and balanced."

Back Relaxer

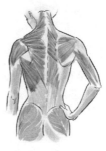

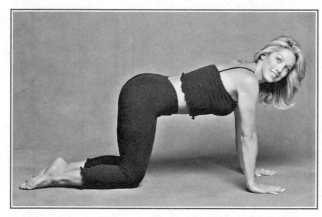

A. Get on your hands and knees, with your abs tight and your back flat. Your hands should be directly under your shoulders and your knees directly under your hips, with the tops of your feet flat on the floor.

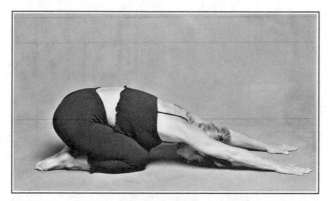

B. From your belly, move your hips back, bringing your buttocks onto the tops of your heels and resting your belly on your thighs. Keep your hands rooted in position throughout the move. Take three deep, cleansing breaths—for about 10 seconds—and then relax. (For cleansing breaths, breathe deeply, fully expanding your lungs and feeling them stretch the back of your ribs. Exhale with a sigh, helping you to sink farther into the stretch.)

Benefit

The back relaxer does just that—it relaxes your back. In this pose, your spine is long. At this point in the sequence, it provides the counterstretch you need after having worked your back muscles during the swimming movement, the Superman, and leg raises.

Pilates Pointers

► When bringing your hips back, pull your belly button in toward your spine. This action will allow you to further extend your buttocks to your heels.

► Keep your shoulder blades spread apart from one another. It should feel as if your thumbs and index fingers want to lift up from the floor, but keep them pressed down.

► Breathe into your ribs, using your breath to expand your back, not your lower belly or chest.

T-Stand

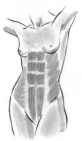

Benefits

Great for the waistline, the T-stand strengthens your arms and shoulders while stretching and strengthening your waist and hips. It also improves your balance.

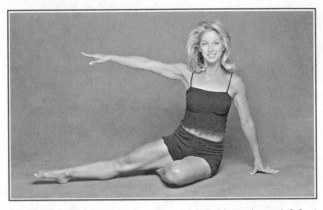

A. Sit with your right leg extended to the side and your left foot tucked in toward your groin area. Extend your right arm out to the side at shoulder level and place your left hand on the floor beside your buttock.

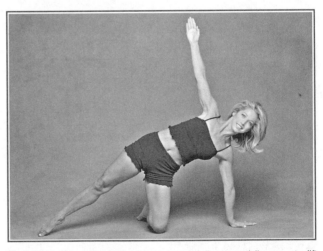

B. Inhale as you use your abs—especially your obliques—to lift your right hip from the floor straight toward the ceiling, as shown, sweeping your right arm up toward the ceiling and pointing your right foot. Your wrist and shoulder should be in a straight line. Also, your wrist should be in a straight line with your knee. Exhale as you lower. Repeat two more times on your right side. Then repeat on the opposite side.

T-Stand

With twist—more challenging

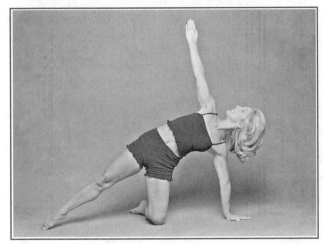

A. Sit with your right leg extended to the side and your left foot tucked in toward your groin area. Extend your right arm out at shoulder level and place your left hand on the floor beside your buttock. Inhale and use your abs to lift your right hip from the floor straight toward the ceiling, as shown, sweeping your right arm up toward the ceiling and pointing your right foot.

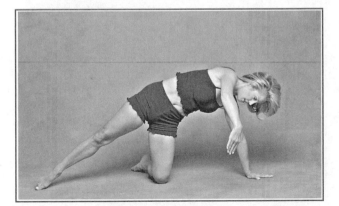

B. Exhale as you slowly sweep your right arm forward, extending through your waist and back.

Pilates Pointers

► Keep your entire body strong while in the raised position.

► Feel yourself reaching up, then feel your upper back stretch.

► When doing the advanced T-stand, shown on page 88, make sure your hips are stacked on top of each other.

—continued

T-Stand

With twist—more challenging—continued

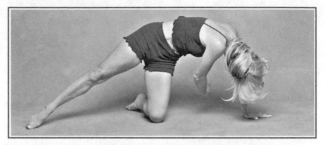

C. Inhale as you reach your right hand under your body and toward your left. Feel your upper back open up, fanning open your upper rib cage. Your obliques and rectus abdominis are working together to keep you up. Then exhale and use your abs to unfold and raise your torso to the starting position. Repeat two more times on your right side. Then repeat on the opposite side.

Advanced T-stand— even more challenging

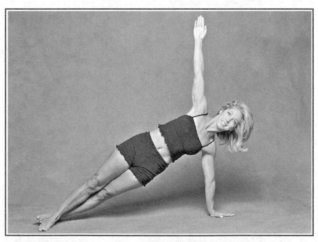

From the sitting position, extend both legs to your right. Then use your abs as you inhale and press through your left hand and lift through your right hip, as shown. You should form the letter T. Hold for 6 to 8 seconds as you inhale and exhale, using percussion breathing if needed. Relax and repeat once more. Then repeat on the opposite side.

Seated Spinal Twist

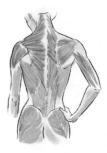

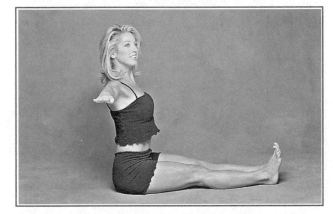

A. Sit with your legs extended and feet flexed. Extend your arms to the sides at shoulder height. Contract your abs to support your back. Your thighs should be working, too. You should be sitting on your sit bones.

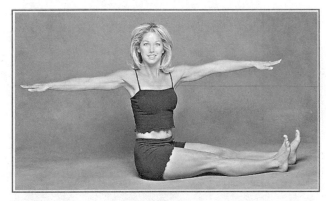

B. Moving from your rib cage, inhale as you rotate toward your right, keeping your back flat and extended. Keep your shoulder blades down toward your hips. Turn your head as you rotate your shoulders. Hold for 1 second then exhale as you face center. Inhale as you repeat by moving to the left. Then repeat on each side once more. During the second stretch, try to rotate just a little farther than before.

Benefits

Rotating the spine is healthy. It keeps the spine lubricated, and it increases circulation to the vertebrae. This move also teaches you to use your abs to lift out of your hips, creating length in your spine. You should be fully warmed up before rotating your back. That's why we always do spinal twists toward the middle to end of a routine.

Pilates Pointers

► Lift out of your hips by pulling in and up with your abs.

► Keep your shoulders down, away from your ears.

► Keep your hips motionless and your buttocks on the floor throughout the move.

► Keep your feet flexed throughout the move, pressing energy out through your heels.

Side Leg Lift

Benefits

Strengthens your obliques, hips, buttocks, and thighs, as well as stretches your inner thighs. It's great for slimming your hips, too!

Pilates Pointers

► Resist the urge to roll your leg inward or to allow your top hip to collapse forward.

► If you must bend your leg, you're lifting too high. Only go as far as you can keep your leg extended.

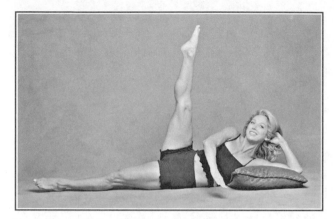

Lie on your left side, with your legs extended, toes pointed, and your left arm supported by a pillow or cushion. Use your left hand to cradle your head and rest your right hand on the floor near your chest. Press your abs toward your spine. With your right leg slightly turned out, inhale as you raise your right leg toward the ceiling, as shown. Exhale as you slowly lower your leg back to the start. Repeat six to eight times and then switch sides.

More challenging

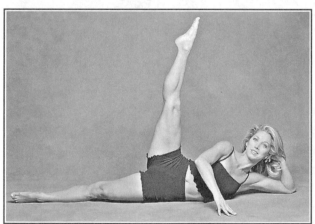

Do the same as the first move but graduate from using the pillow or cushion for support.

Denise-eology . . .

"Remember, the core stays strong, yet still."

Side Leg Circles

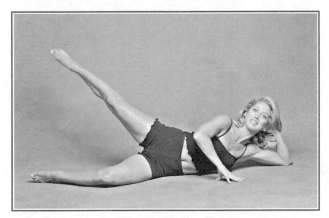

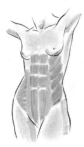

Lie on your left side, supporting your head in your left hand. Bend your left leg for support and rest your right hand on the floor near your chest. Point your right foot and extend through your right leg, raising it only as high as you can keep your abs tight and hips stacked on top of each other. Then draw small clockwise circles with your right big toe, trying to initiate the motion from your hip joint and keeping your abs strong throughout. Breathe normally. Draw five circles and then reverse the direction. Switch sides and repeat.

More challenging

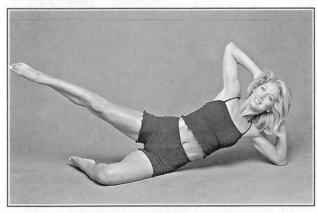

Do the same as the regular leg circles, but this time lift your torso off the floor, working your obliques (your waistline) as you do so.

Benefits

This move works those trouble spots (the hips, buttocks, and thighs) as well as the powerhouse (your abs, waistline, and entire torso).

Pilates Pointers

► Keep your top leg long, extending all the way from your hip to your big toe.

► Use your abs to keep your hips in line, not allowing your body to sink forward.

Denise-eology . . .

"Reshape your thighs to a perfect size. All the strength without the bulk."

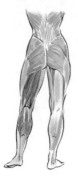

Front/Back

Benefits

This move stretches your thighs; strengthens your lower back, hips, and buttocks; and challenges you to stabilize your hips during movement.

Pilates Pointers

▶ Think "long" throughout the move. Push through your feet and the crown of your head to make your body as long as possible.

▶ Use the strength of your abs to keep your hips stacked on top of each other and stable throughout the move. Don't let your top hip lean back or forward.

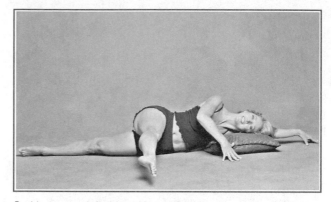

A. Lie on your left side, with your head supported by a pillow or cushion and your left arm extended above your head behind the pillow. Extend both legs on top of each other with your toes pointed. Bring your legs slightly in front of the plane of your body and turn your left leg toward the floor for support. Contract your abs and inhale as you slowly kick your right leg forward, as shown, keeping your left leg and foot pressed into the floor.

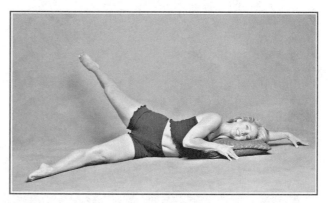

B. Once you've swept your leg as far forward as you can, exhale as you sweep it back, behind your body and slightly up. Keep your abs strong throughout and squeeze your buttocks. Repeat six to eight times and then switch sides.

Grande Ronde de Jambe

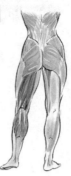

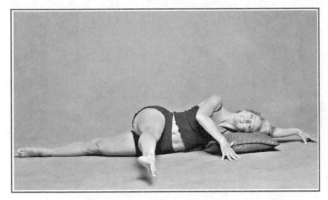

A. Begin in the front/back position on your left side with your right leg extended from your hip at a 90-degree angle from your torso and hovering just an inch from the floor.

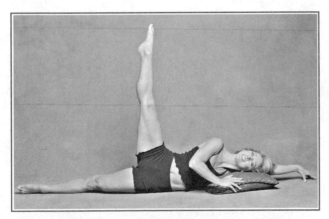

B. Press your abs to your spine, elongate your body, and inhale as you rotate your right leg up, moving from the hip socket. Point your toes to the ceiling.

Benefits

This means "large leg circle" in French. It stretches your thighs; strengthens your lower back, hips, and buttocks; and challenges you to stabilize your hips during movement.

Pilates Pointer

▶ Keep your abs, torso, and back stable as you move your leg.

Denise-eology . . .

"Feel like a ballerina with those beautiful, long, lean legs. You will see results."

—continued

Grande Ronde de Jambe
—continued

Denise-eology . . .
"You can't change your bone structure— your skeleton— but you can change your fat content and muscle tone."

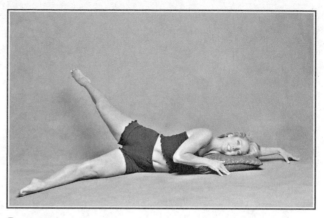

C. Exhale and reach your right leg behind you, as shown, keeping your abs tight and hips stable. Then inhale as you swing your leg to the front and repeat the sequence two more times. Reverse the direction for three circles, then switch sides and repeat the sequence.

Single-Leg Teaser

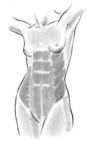

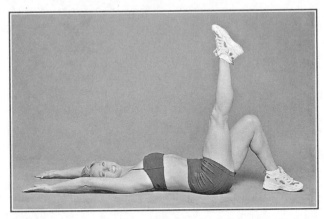

A. Lie on your back with your arms extended overhead, your left knee bent, and your right leg extended at a 90-degree angle from your hip.

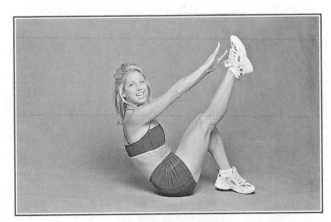

B. Exhale as you use your abs to curl your upper body up toward your extended leg and as you simultaneously lower your arms to chest level and extend them toward your right foot. Hold for 2 seconds, inhaling and exhaling. Then exhale as you lower to the starting position. Repeat one time, then switch to the other leg for two repetitions.

Benefits

This strengthens your core, readying you for the teaser (on page 96). It will teach you to keep your abs tight as you move continuously. Plus, it's great for the lower abs.

Pilates Pointers

► As you rise, try not to press into the foot that's on the floor. Use your abs to do all of the work.

► Keep your shoulder blades pressed down, away from your ears. Also, keep them pressed back, opening your chest.

► Try to keep your abs and your ribs in a flat line throughout the move.

► Keep your knees pressed together at the top of the move.

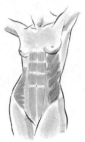

Teaser

Benefits

One of the most advanced Pilates moves, the teaser completely tests your abdominal strength and balance. It's the ultimate challenge and my personal secret for strong, flat abs.

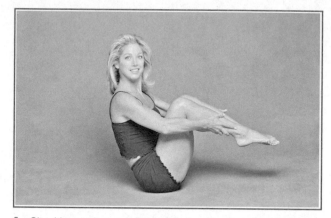

A. Sit with your knees bent and feet on the floor. Hold on to your calves with your hands as you slowly sit back, bring your feet a couple of inches off the floor, and balance on your sit bones. Inhale.

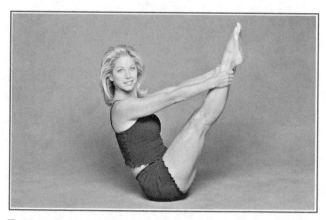

B. Exhale as you press your abs toward your spine and extend your legs and point your toes, only using your hands slightly to keep your upper body in position. Inhale. Hold the position for 2 seconds, then exhale as you lower. Repeat two times.

Teaser

Most challenging

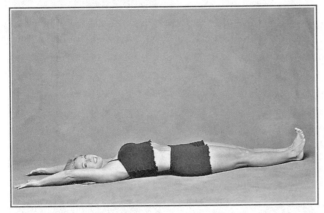

A. Lie on your back with your arms extended over your head, your legs extended. Lengthen your body by pressing through your heels and fingertips, but keep your abs pressed toward your spine.

Pilates Pointers

► Keep your shoulders relaxed, with your shoulder blades pressed down and back to open your chest.

► Try to scoop in your abs to keep your back flat.

► Extend through your toes and the crown of your head.

► Do the best you can. This one is very challenging, so you only need to do it two times . . . it's that effective.

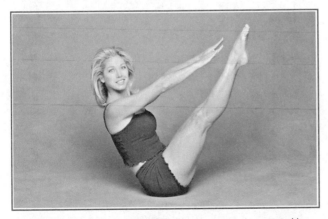

B. Exhale as you simultaneously lift your arms, torso, and legs to form a V shape with your body and point your toes. Press your abs toward your spine throughout the move and squeeze through your inner thighs. Inhale. Hold the position for 2 seconds. Exhale as you slowly lower to the starting position. Repeat two times.

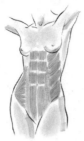

Shoulder Stand

Challenging

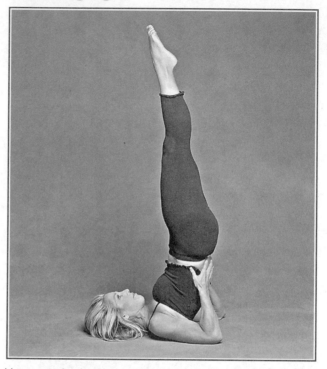

Benefits

The preceding moves have completely stretched and strengthened your entire body. Now is the perfect time to work every muscle in your body in a shoulder stand. The shoulder stand strengthens your abs; stretches your back, shoulders, and neck; and revitalizes your body with fresh oxygen and blood. Upside-down poses reverse the effects of gravity, making you feel focused and energized.

Note: Because you're in an upside-down position, do not perform this move if you have a neck or back problem or high blood pressure.

Lie on your back with your knees pulled in toward your chest and your hands on the floor at hip level. In one fluid motion, inhale as you use your abs to roll your buttocks into the air and straighten your legs. (As you gain abdominal strength, you'll be able to jackknife straightened legs into the air. You won't need to bend them first.)

With your elbows close to your torso, walk your hands up your back, using your hands and the strength in your abs to pull your back and legs into a straight, vertical line, as shown. Imagine that a string is gently pulling your big toes toward the ceiling. Keep your body weight over your shoulders and arms, not on your neck and head. Breathe deeply, exhaling and inhaling, and hold for 10 to 30 seconds, lower, and repeat once.

Shoulder Stand

With scissors—more challenging

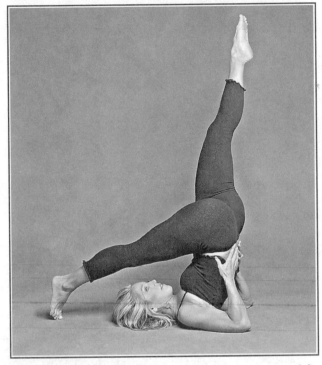

From the shoulder stand position, exhale as you lower your left leg toward the floor behind your head. Your left knee should be in line with your eyes. Inhale as you raise your leg back to its vertical position. Then repeat with your right leg, exhaling as you lower it, inhaling as you raise it. Continue alternating your legs, repeating the sequence four more times.

Denise-eology . . .

"Challenge your pessimistic thoughts by visualizing yourself doing the unthinkable."

Pilates Pointers

► Stick with the regular shoulder stand, on the opposite page, until you can fully extend and flatten your back, with your hips and feet directly above your shoulders.

► When you bring your leg back behind your head, make sure to keep your back flat and extended directly above your shoulders. Don't slide your hips behind or in front of your shoulders. Also, don't round your back. Use your abs to hold your back in position.

► While in this pose, do not turn your head out of position.

► Focus on contracting your hipbones toward your ribs. This will help keep your back flat.

► Don't forget to breathe deeply and normally.

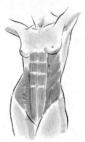

Leg Pull Back

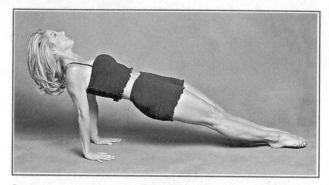

Benefits

This stretches your hamstrings, builds leg strength, firms your buttocks, works the deepest layer of your abs, and challenges you to keep your shoulders in the correct position.

Pilates Pointers

► Imagine balancing a plate on your chest and your abdomen. Don't let it fall off!

► Balance on the center of your heel. Keep your supporting leg strong. Use your quadriceps (the muscles that form the front of your thighs) to pull your kneecap up, preventing your leg from hyperextending.

► This isn't a contest to see how high you can raise your leg. Raise it no higher than you can keep your entire body in a straight line.

A. Sit on the floor with your legs extended in front of you and your hands pressed into the floor next to your buttocks. Contract your abs as you exhale and press into your palms, straightening your arms and body, as shown. Your forehead, shoulders, hips, and heels should form a straight line. Make sure your shoulder blades are pushed back and low on your back, so that your chest is open and your neck is long. Imagine that a string is lifting your chest toward the ceiling.

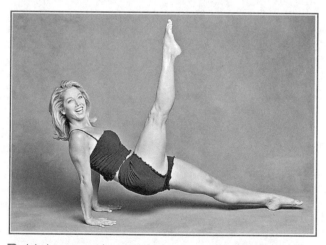

B. Inhale as you raise your right leg up, using the strength of your abs to keep your hips level, and press up toward the ceiling. Exhale as you slowly lower your leg. Switch legs and repeat. Continue alternating your legs, repeating the sequence two more times, then relax.

Leg Pull Front

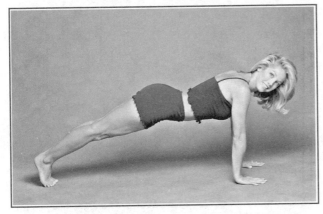

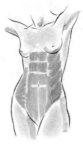

A. Get in a standard pushup position with your palms on the floor under your chest, your legs extended, and your weight on the balls of your feet. Contract your abs so that your back doesn't arch or your buttocks don't sink down below the plane of your body. Your body should form a straight line from your heels to your head.

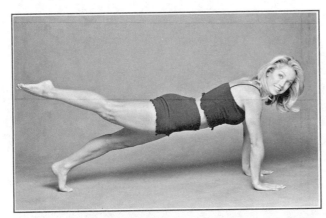

B. Inhale as you raise your right leg up as high as you can behind you without arching your lower back or allowing your hips to fall out of alignment. Exhale as you lower your leg to the starting position. Repeat with the left leg. Continue alternating your legs, repeating the sequence two more times.

Benefits

Strengthens your abdomen and lengthens from your hip joints, preventing lower back problems. This is great for stabilizing your powerhouse and strengthening your entire body.

Pilates Pointers

▶ Try to form a straight line with your body.

▶ Lengthen through the crown of your head to keep your shoulders from slouching.

▶ Keep your hips level. Don't fall out to one side.

▶ Keep your body weight between your big and second toes.

▶ As you raise your leg, imagine the motion starting in your abs, not from your foot.

▶ Focus on your abs—pull them up and in.

Leg Pull Front

More challenging

Pilates Pointer

► Tucking your tummy up toward your spine will help you to keep your hips level and motionless throughout this move. It will also help with your balance.

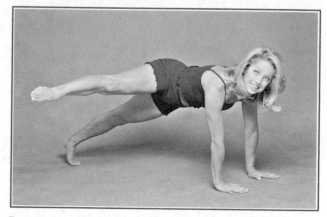

From the same starting position, raise your right leg up and to the right. This takes more balance and abdominal strength to keep your hips level. Try two on each side.

Denise-eology . . .

"You should feel proud of yourself; you're doing great."

Pilates Pushup

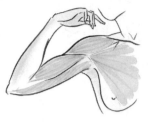

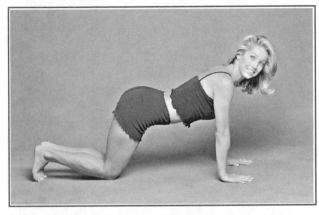

A. Get on all fours, with your knees under your hips and your hands under your chest.

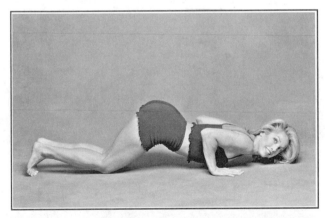

B. Press your abs against your spine as you inhale and slowly lower your chest to the floor, as shown, keeping your arms close to your torso and your back flat. Exhale as you press through your knees and your hands to rise to the starting position. Perform three to five perfect pushups and then relax.

Benefits

As with regular pushups, these strengthen your chest, upper arms, shoulders, and upper back. Unlike regular pushups, they also help you move from your powerhouse, developing your inner strength.

Pilates Pointers

► Keep your elbows close to your sides throughout the move.

► Keep your abs strong to prevent your hips from sinking.

Pilates Pushup

More challenging

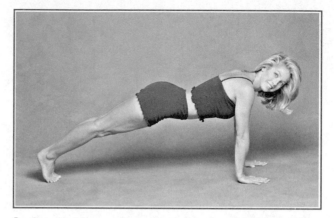

A. Get on all fours, with your knees under your hips and your hands under your chest. Extend your legs so you are balancing on the balls of your feet and your body is extended from your feet to your head, as shown. Make sure that your abs are engaged.

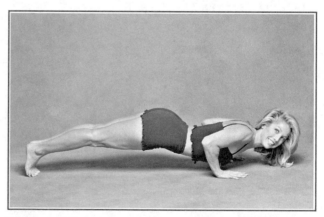

B. Inhale as you slowly lower your chest toward the floor, making sure to move from your abs, not your arms. Once you reach the floor, activate your abs to rise back to the starting position as you exhale. Perform three to five perfect pushups and then relax.

Child's Pose

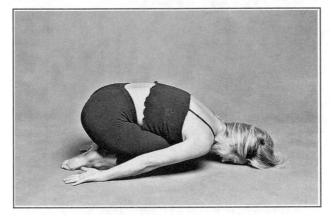

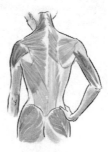

Get on all fours with your knees under your hips and your hands under your shoulders. Pull your tummy against your spine as you bring your buttocks back toward your heels. Once your torso rests on your thighs, lower your forehead to the floor and turn it to the side for comfort. Then slide your arms along the floor and bring them behind your body, as shown, palms facing the ceiling. Take three deep, cleansing breaths and then relax.

Benefits

A wonderful way to relax your back, this pose lengthens your spine, stretches your entire back, and gives you a deep, comfortable rest.

Pilates Pointer

► Pulling your belly button against your spine will allow you to bring your tailbone closer to your heels.

Denise-eology . . .

"This is my favorite stretch of all. Inhale energy, and exhale any tension."

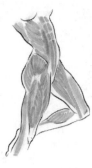

Downward Facing Dog

Benefits

Talk about a move that simultaneously stretches and strengthens nearly the entire body! My favorite pose from yoga, I put a Pilates emphasis on this one.

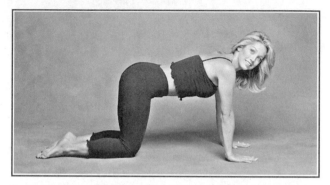

A. From all fours, with your hands under your shoulders and your knees under your hips, pull your navel toward your spine as you exhale and press back through your palms and bring your buttocks close to your heels.

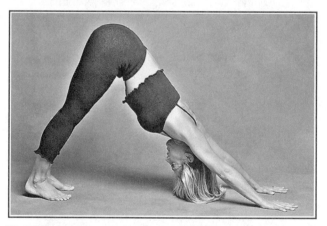

B. Bring the balls of your feet onto the floor, and, keeping your navel pressed against your spine, inhale and raise your tailbone toward the ceiling, as shown. Eventually, you'll want to press your heels toward the floor, but you may not at first have the flexibility to do so. In that case, start with your knees slightly bent, concentrating on pressing your tailbone to the sky and scooping your abs toward your spine. Slowly try to straighten your legs. Take three deep, cleansing breaths and then relax.

Downward Facing Dog

More challenging

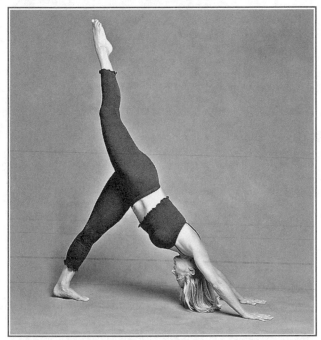

Once you can lower your heels close to the floor without losing the scoop in your abs or your long, flat back, you're ready for the advanced pose. From the downward facing dog position, shift your body weight onto your left foot, and, while keeping your hips level, raise your right leg up, as shown. At first you may not be able to fully extend your right leg. That's fine. Allow your calf to stretch as you concentrate on keeping your belly pressed against your spine and keeping your hips level. Visualize bringing your right hipbone down and forward while pushing your left hipbone back and up. Take three deep, cleansing breaths and switch legs. Then come back to the downward facing dog position with both legs together and then relax.

Pilates Pointers

► When coming into the pose, move first from your hips, not from your head. Curling your belly against your spine and raising your hips up will automatically bring your head into position.

► Relax your head and neck. Gaze at your navel during the pose.

► Keep your shoulders in position. Pull your shoulder blades away from your ears and roll them away from each other, creating more width in your upper back.

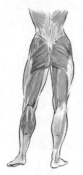

Forward Bend

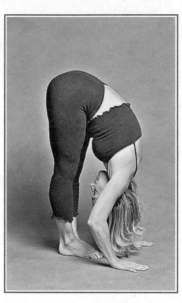

Benefits

Stretches and strengthens your hamstrings as well as stretches your back.

Pilates Pointers

► If your belly and legs are not strong enough to hold your body weight, bend your knees as you bend forward and slide your hands against your legs for support.

► Keep the emphasis on pressing your belly button toward your spine. That may mean you can't bend as far forward. Remember, this isn't a flexibility contest.

► Keep your knees slightly bent throughout the move to prevent hyperextending your knee joint.

► Relax your neck muscles, let your head hang down, and let gravity create space between each vertebra.

From the downward facing dog position, walk your hands back toward your toes. Bend your knees if you have to, ensuring that your back is flat. Your tailbone to your midback should form a flat line. Press your abs to your spine. Hold the stretch for three deep, cleansing breaths, then relax.

Denise-eology . . .
"You are as young as you feel. Keep your back strong and healthy."

Full-Body Reach-Up

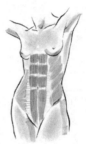

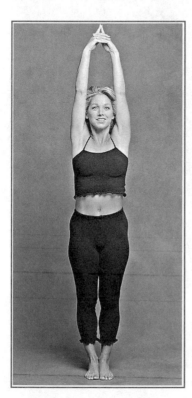

A. From the forward bend, press your belly button to your spine and, starting with your lower abs, roll up, one vertebra at a time, bringing your shoulders, neck, then head up last. Stand with your ankles and inner thighs pressed together and your abs engaged. Raise your arms above your head and bring them together in a temple pose, as shown, with your index fingers extended, pressing through your index fingers to create length in your body. Keep your shoulders relaxed.

Benefits

Stretches and strengthens the sides of your back and abdomen.

Pilates Pointers

► Keep your abs pressed against your spine throughout the move.

► Don't allow your top hip to roll forward. Keep your chest open.

—continued

Full-Body Reach-Up

—continued

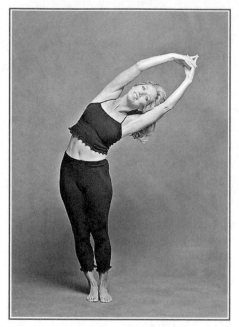

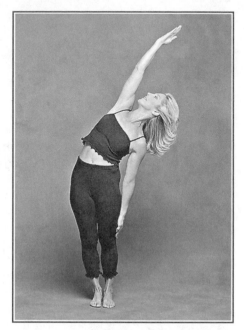

B. Keeping your abs pressed against your spine, inhale and exhale as you bend to the left, leading with your index fingers. Keep your hipbones level with one another.

C. Lower your left arm to your outer left thigh and reach up and over with your right hand, as shown, feeling a deep stretch from your outer right thigh all the way to your fingertips. Gaze at the ceiling to bring the stretch through the front of your neck. Inhale as you rise to center, bringing your hands together in a temple pose. Exhale as you bend to the right and complete the sequence. Repeat one more time on each side.

Chest Expansion

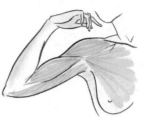

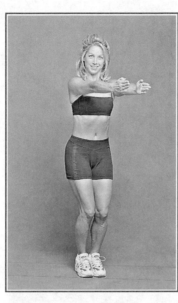

Benefits

This stretches and opens the chest, making breathing easier and relieving tension.

Pilates Pointers

► Keep a slight bend in your knees.

► Imagine a string connecting your breastbone to the ceiling. Let that string pull your breastbone up, expanding your chest.

► Roll your armpits out, opening your chest even more.

A. Stand with your knees slightly bent and your tummy tight. Extend your arms in front of you so that your hands are at shoulder level, with your palms facing each other.

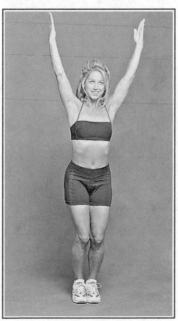

B. Extend your arms overhead, opening your chest. Don't let your abs collapse, as this will collapse your chest as well. Breathe deeply as your chest opens. Hold the stretch as you inhale and exhale for three deep, cleansing breaths, then relax.

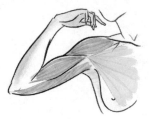

Chest Lift

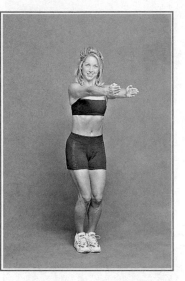

Benefits

Stretching and opening your chest will improve your posture and help you move your upper body more fluidly.

Pilates Pointers

► As you extend your arms to the sides, don't hunch your shoulders toward your ears. Instead, keep your shoulder blades pressed down.

► Keep your head above your shoulders, so that your chin is not jutting forward.

A. Stand with your knees slightly bent and your tummy tight. Extend your arms in front of you so that your hands are at shoulder level, with your palms facing each other.

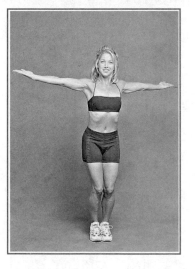

B. Open your arms to the sides, slightly behind your body if you can, with your palms up. Breathe deeply as your chest opens. Hold the stretch as you inhale and exhale for three deep, cleansing breaths, then relax.

Alternating Arms Scissors

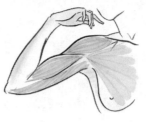

Stand with your knees slightly bent, your abs engaged, and your arms extended in front of you at chest level, as shown. Take in a deep breath. Now exhale as you press through your fingers and raise your right hand up above your head and your left arm down toward your feet. Then switch, raising your left hand as you lower your right arm. Continue alternating your arms, repeating the sequence four more times.

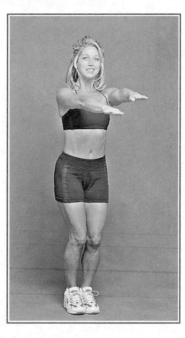

Benefits

This move will stretch your chest muscles, which in turn will improve your upper back and neck posture.

Pilates Pointers

► Do this move in front of a mirror to ensure that you don't arch your back.

► Press through your fingertips for length, as if you had strings attached to both index fingers and someone were pulling one hand toward the floor and the other toward the ceiling.

THE Complete Pilates PROGRAM at a Glance

The Complete Pilates Program follows a sequential order that allows you to flow through the workout. You may need to build strength and flexibility, however, before you can complete this entire sequence without resting. If you need to rest between challenging poses, bring your body into the child's pose.

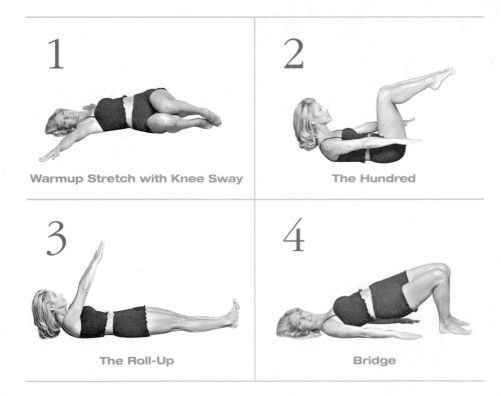

1

Warmup Stretch with Knee Sway

2

The Hundred

3

The Roll-Up

4

Bridge

114   The Core Movements

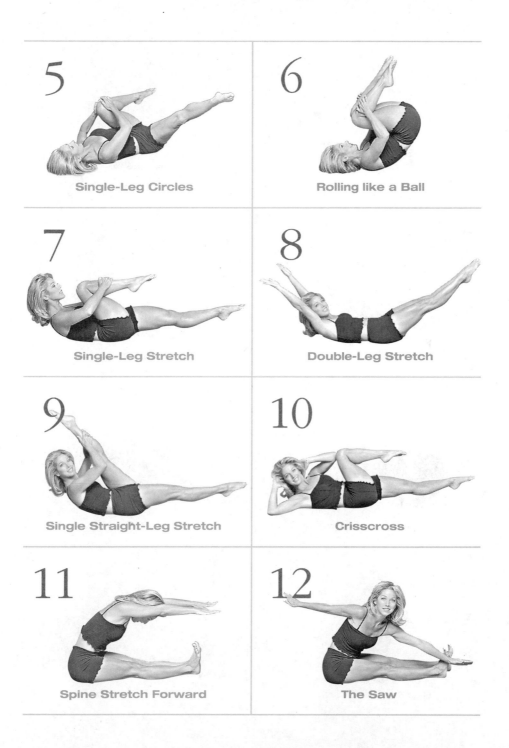

5 Single-Leg Circles

6 Rolling like a Ball

7 Single-Leg Stretch

8 Double-Leg Stretch

9 Single Straight-Leg Stretch

10 Crisscross

11 Spine Stretch Forward

12 The Saw

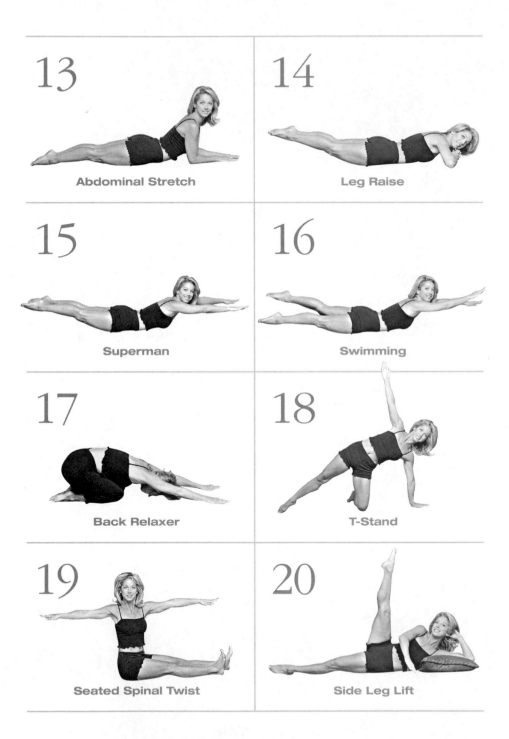

13 Abdominal Stretch

14 Leg Raise

15 Superman

16 Swimming

17 Back Relaxer

18 T-Stand

19 Seated Spinal Twist

20 Side Leg Lift

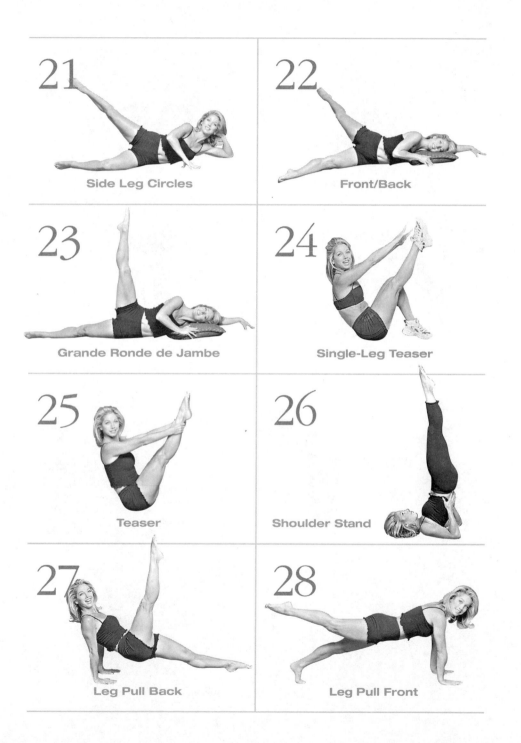

21 Side Leg Circles

22 Front/Back

23 Grande Ronde de Jambe

24 Single-Leg Teaser

25 Teaser

26 Shoulder Stand

27 Leg Pull Back

28 Leg Pull Front

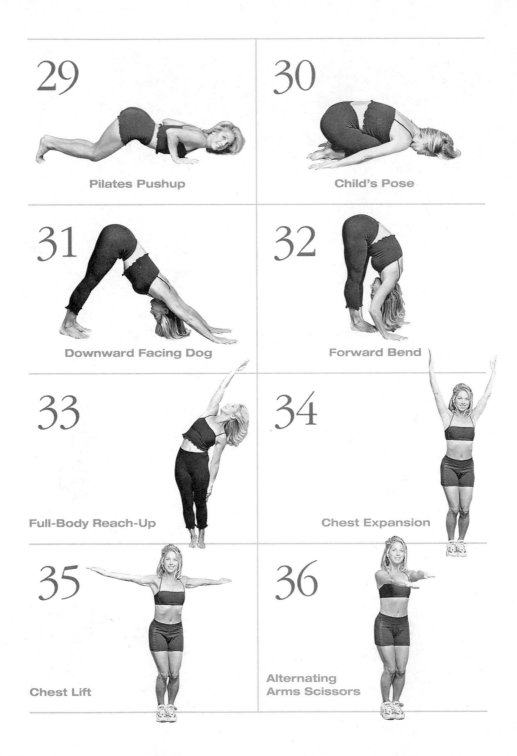

29 Pilates Pushup

30 Child's Pose

31 Downward Facing Dog

32 Forward Bend

33 Full-Body Reach-Up

34 Chest Expansion

35 Chest Lift

36 Alternating Arms Scissors

The WARMUP and COOLDOWN Program

This routine stretches all of your muscles, from your feet to your head. To keep your body pliable and flexible for Pilates moves, practice these stretches before or after any Pilates routine, be it the Beginner Program, the Complete Program, one of the 5- or 10-minute routines in part 3, or the three-times-a-week Pilates sessions in part 4. These are also great stretches to do after any aerobic activity—such as walking, running, or the in-home cardio program in part 4—because they will lengthen any muscles that may have tightened during your workout, preventing post-exercise stiffness.

I also like to do these stretches any time I've been sitting for a long time or when I am generally feeling tight or achy. They loosen up stiff muscles and get blood circulating to the joints. Do them whenever you need a break, need some extra energy, or just want to feel good. They truly feel fantastic—and they take only 10 minutes of your time.

As with the other routines in this section, these stretches flow in a sequential order. Each stretch prepares you for the one that comes next. Hold each stretch for at least 10 seconds. If you can hold for 20, that's even better. Relax during the stretch by breathing slowly and deeply. Don't bounce. Just give in. Feel the stretch, but don't overdo it. Aim for length, not pain.

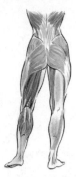

Hip/Buttocks Stretch

Benefits

This stretches your hips, buttocks, and lower back and feels wonderful! Also, this hip/buttocks stretch helps relieve lower back tension by keeping your hips and buttock muscles flexible.

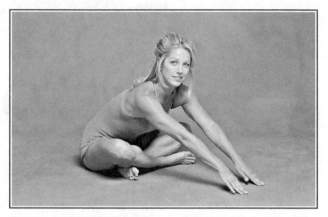

A. Sit comfortably with your legs crossed. Lengthen through the crown of your head as you press your abs against your spine. Keeping your abs pressed against your spine, bend forward from your hips, reaching forward with your fingertips, as shown. You'll feel the stretch along the outer thigh, butt cheek, and hip of whichever leg is in front. Breathe deeply as your hip relaxes.

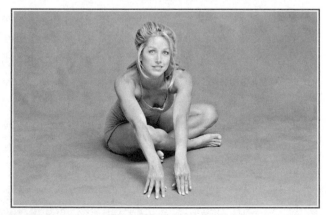

B. Keeping your abs pressed against your spine, slowly move your chest toward the right, continuing to reach through your fingertips. This will give you a deeper stretch in your lower back and hips. Breathe deeply as your hip relaxes.

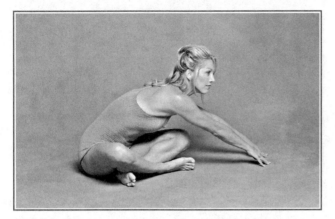

C. Slowly reach through your fingertips as you move your chest to the left. Breathe deeply as your hip relaxes. Bring your arms back to center and rise to the starting position. Switch your legs so the other leg is in front and repeat the sequence.

Pilates Pointers

► If you keep your abs pressed against your spine, you won't be able to bend as far forward as you would if you let them relax, but you'll achieve a deeper stretch.

► Keep your back flat by bending from your hips, not from your middle or upper back.

Denise-eology . . .

"As we age, we lose elasticity— unless we stretch. These stretches will keep you moving with grace."

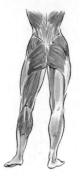

Leg Stretch

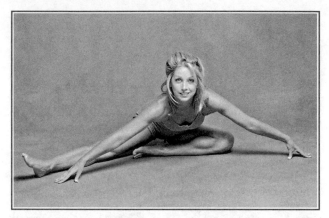

Sit with your left leg bent and left foot pulled close to your groin area. Extend your right leg at a 45-degree angle from your torso. Pull your abs toward your spine as you exhale and bend forward, as shown, feeling the stretch along the inner and back thigh of your extended leg. Switch legs and repeat the sequence.

Benefits

Great for keeping your back healthy, this move stretches the backs of your thighs as well as your inner thighs.

Pilates Pointers

► Remember to keep your abs pressed against your spine.

► Take your time.

► Try to keep your buttocks on the floor.

Denise-eology . . .

"Flexibility takes regular effort . . . so keep it up."

Spinal Twist

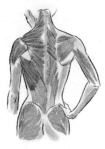

A. Sit with your legs extended in front of you. Bend your left knee and pull your left heel in toward your right buttock. Bend your right knee and place your right foot just to the outside of your left knee, as shown. Your legs should resemble a pretzel shape.

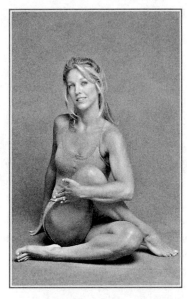

B. Sit tall, lengthening through your crown and pulling your abs toward your spine as you inhale and rotate to the right. Use your right hand to press into the floor and keep your body upright, as shown, not leaning back. To rotate a little farther, use your left hand to gently pull your thigh. Exhale and release. Repeat on the other side, rearranging your legs so that your left leg is on top.

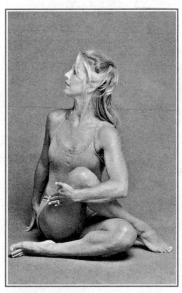

Benefits

This movement stretches your hips and stretches and rotates your spine, ribs, and abdomen.

Pilates Pointers

► Move from your hips up, not from your shoulders down. Imagine that your spine is a straight pole and you are rotating your body around that pole.

► Use the strength in your abs to increase your rotation.

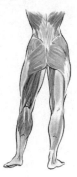

Hip Opener

Benefits

Stretches your buttocks, hips, hip flexors (in your pelvis), quadriceps (the muscles that form the front of your thighs), lower back, and outer thighs, preventing back pain. It's great for women—our hip sockets are different from men's, giving us tighter hip muscles. Though you may feel tight in this stretch, once you surrender to it, it feels wonderful.

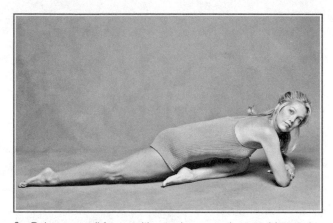

A. Balance on all fours, with your knees under your hips and your hands under your shoulders. Bring your left knee in toward your chest, resting your outer left shin and outer left thigh on the floor. Extend your right leg straight back. Bend your arms, as shown, and support your body weight with your forearms as your hip opens. Breathe deeply as your hip relaxes.

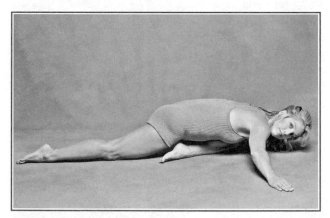

B. Once your hip opens and your left buttock moves closer to the floor, extend your arms to the sides, as shown, placing most of your body weight over your bent leg. Your body weight will force your hip to open even more. Don't try this if you still feel uncomfortable in the basic position. Breathe deeply as your hip relaxes. Repeat with the other leg.

Hip Opener

More challenging

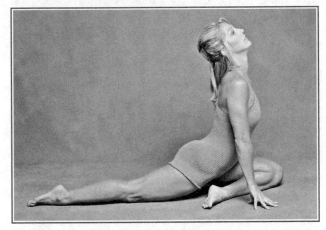

Press your navel in against your spine to pull your left buttock as close to the floor as possible. Press through your hands and raise your chest, as shown, opening it toward the ceiling. If you're working your abs correctly, you should have very little body weight on your hands.

Pilates Pointers

► Allow your lower back to widen as you sink into this stretch.

► Use your abs to increase the stretch and prevent pinching or strain in your lower back.

► Try to keep your hips level.

Denise-eology . . .

"Judge your success not by financial gain, but by the degree to which you are enjoying health, peace, and love. These commodities can never be traded or bartered."

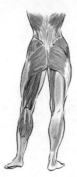

Benefits

This opens the hips and stretches the large gluteal muscles in your backside.

Pilates Pointers

► Maintain control and engage your abs during the stretch.

► Pulling your tailbone toward the floor will help increase your flexibility.

► Another way to really feel the stretch is to slowly rock side to side to target the hamstring muscle that goes through your buttocks.

Denise's Favorite Lower Body Stretch

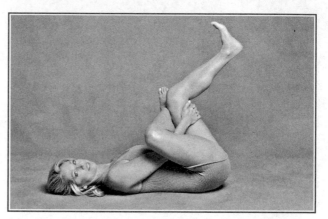

Lie on your back with your knees bent and feet flat on the floor. Raise your right knee and place your outer right shin on top of your left lower thigh, just above your left knee. Pull your abs toward your spine as you lift your left knee toward your chest. Reach your hands around your left thigh (threading your right arm through the triangle of space between your legs) and gently pull it closer to your chest, as shown. Breathe deeply as your hip relaxes. Repeat with the other leg.

Back and Hamstring Stretch

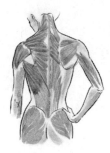

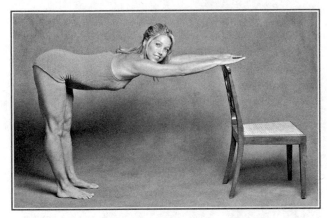

Stand 2 to 3 feet away from a chair. Reach your arms overhead and bend forward from your hips, controlling your forward movement with the strength of your abs. When your hands reach the top of the chair, rest them there, as shown. If your feet are in front of your hips, move them back. Then breathe deeply as you stretch back through your tailbone.

Benefit

This classic stretch lengthens your entire spine, from your neck to your tailbone, and stretches the backs of your legs.

Pilates Pointer

► Imagine that a high-strength magnet is pulling your tailbone toward the wall behind you.

Denise-eology . . .

"Streamline your body and use your breath to relax you so that your energy will flow from the inside out."

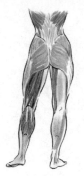

Buttocks Stretch

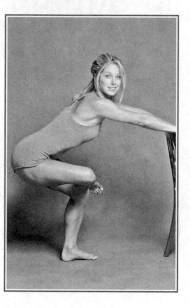

Benefits

This move stretches your hips and buttocks while simultaneously improving your balance.

Pilates Pointer

▶ Your abs help you balance. If you feel wobbly, focus on your center and steady yourself from your core.

Stand 2 to 3 feet in front of a chair. Place your right ankle on your lower left thigh, just above the knee. Reach forward and place both hands on the back of the chair, as shown, for balance as you slowly bend your left knee. Once your knee bends, your right leg will stay put. Breathe deeply as your hip joint opens. Repeat with the other leg.

More challenging

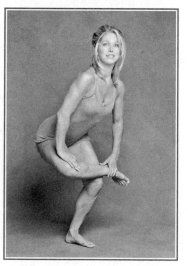

If you feel balanced and flexible in the beginner pose, try it without the chair. As you bend your leg, keep your back flat and your abs pressed against your spine.

Calf Stretch

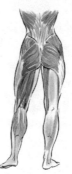

Stand a foot away from a chair. Rest your hands on the top of the chair and take a large step back with your right leg. Bend your left knee and extend back through your right heel, feeling a stretch in your right calf. Breathe deeply as your calf relaxes. Repeat with the other leg.

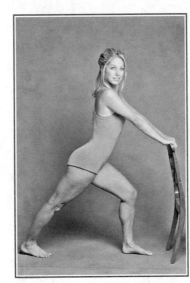

Benefit

A favorite with runners, this is an excellent stretch for your calf muscles, which prevents tightness.

Pilates Pointers

► Stay upright during this stretch. Don't lean too far forward.

► Pulling your abs toward your spine will increase the stretch in your rear leg.

Denise-eology . . .

"If you wear shoes with heels that are 2 inches or higher, you need to stretch your calves. If you don't, the tightness in your lower legs can tug on your lower back."

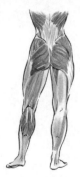

Thigh Stretch

Benefits

Great for leg circulation, this stretches the backs of your thighs, your inner thighs, your hips, and your lower back.

Pilates Pointers

► Keep your abs engaged and your shoulders relaxed.

► Use your abs at your waist to pull your leg higher.

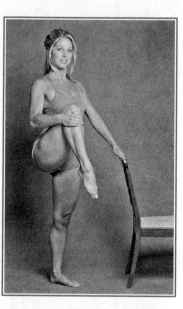

A. Stand next to a chair. Place your body weight onto your left foot and raise your right knee toward your chest. Use the chair for balance, if needed. Wrap your fingers around your right shin to pull your leg a little higher, increasing the stretch. Breathe deeply as your thigh relaxes.

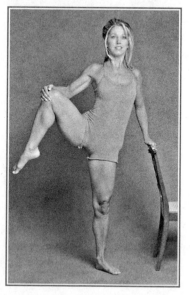

B. Rotate your right thigh to the right, feeling a stretch along your inner thigh. Breathe deeply as your thigh relaxes. Return to the starting position and repeat with the other leg.

Quad/Hip Flexor Stretch

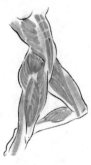

Stand a foot away from a chair. Place your body weight onto your left foot. Bend your right knee, bringing your right foot toward your buttocks. Grasp your right ankle with your right hand, as shown. Pull your abs to your spine and focus on extending your right knee down, toward the floor. Breathe deeply as your thigh relaxes. Repeat with the other leg.

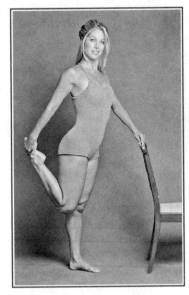

Benefits

Stretches your quadriceps muscles and your hip flexors, which connect the top of the quads through the pelvis to the lower spine.

Pilates Pointers

► Many people do this stretch incorrectly by pulling their knee behind their bodies rather than extending it down. If your abs are truly pulled against your spine, you'll feel a deep stretch to your thigh as you extend your knee down, not back.

► Try to keep your knees together.

Denise-eology . . .

"Just stretch to a comfortable position, especially at the beginning of each stretch, then the 'stretch tension' should slowly subside as you hold it. Keep limber."

THE Warmup AND Cooldown PROGRAM at a Glance

Try this sequence of stretches before or after any of the Pilates routines in this book, or after any aerobic workout or sport, including the cardio workouts in part 4. If you like, you can also do some of these stretches at midmorning or midafternoon to unkink your body after sitting at a computer for hours.

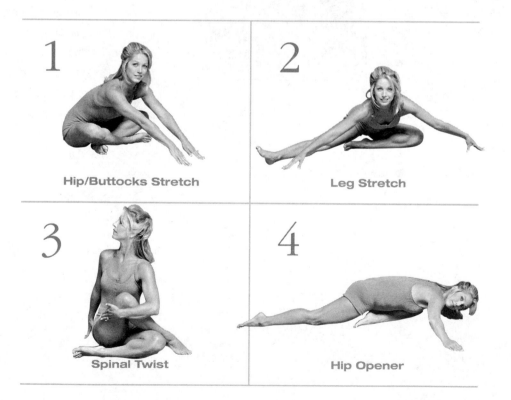

1 Hip/Buttocks Stretch

2 Leg Stretch

3 Spinal Twist

4 Hip Opener

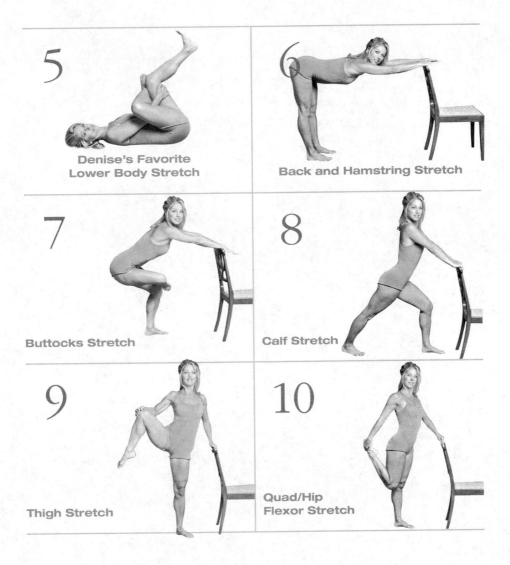

5 Denise's Favorite Lower Body Stretch

6 Back and Hamstring Stretch

7 Buttocks Stretch

8 Calf Stretch

9 Thigh Stretch

10 Quad/Hip Flexor Stretch

Denise-eology . . .

"When you finish a Pilates workout,
you don't simply feel better—
you feel better about yourself."

Part

3

PICK YOUR Plan

SIX Routines, 10 MINUTES at a Time

Do you want to slim your hips or thighs? Do you wish you could tone up that stubborn flab underneath your upper arms? Do you wince at the way your lower belly has pooched out ever since your last pregnancy? Do you have back or joint pain?

If you answered yes to any of those questions, the Pilates routines in this section are for you. Parts 2 and 4 of this book offer you routines for total-body conditioning. Here, I developed routines that target specific trouble spots (such as the tummy, buttocks, and thighs) or accomplish specific goals (such as preventing or relieving joint or lower back pain or getting in shape after having a baby). Each of the following routines will target a particular trouble spot in addition to your core—the abs and back.

If, like me, the race is on from the moment you get out of bed in the morning until you go to bed at night, you'll love these routines because they're short and effective. Each routine lasts no more than 10 minutes. Any given routine gives you the minimum dose required to be fit and flexible. Don't forget to add warmup and cooldown stretches from part 2 before or after each workout.

Pick the routine that you feel you need the most and use it as a wonderful complement to your complete Pilates routine. Do these routines whenever you can squeeze them in. For example, if you have time, add one of these routines to your Complete Pilates Program from part 2. If you don't have a lot of time, consider one of these routines instead of the Complete Pilates Program.

Here's another great idea, which I like to do: Mix and match these routines with your 3-Week Total Body Makeover program in part 4. Once you've finished the 3-Week Total Body Makeover, stick with the Pilates workouts you enjoyed most from that plan and substitute any of these shorter workouts for ones that suit you less.

For example, your goal is to do Pilates three times a week. One day you might do the 10-Minute Upper Body Routine on page 161 in this section. Another day you might tackle the Complete Pilates Program from part 2. A third day you might stick with a Pilates routine from the 3-Week Total Body Makeover.

Mixing and matching routines from throughout the book provides the variety you need to stay motivated. It will also help you work different muscles, keeping your workouts most effective.

You *Can* Find the Time!

No matter how short your exercise routine, you'll only stick with it if you first learn how to balance life's demands and carve out time for yourself. I know. I had to do the same thing.

With two television shows to produce and shoot, I have a busy work schedule. Between getting up, working out, getting the kids up and out the door to school, running errands, straightening the house, doing chores, tending to work-related business, spending time with the kids and my husband, plus making dinner, sometimes it is hard for me to always see what's most important.

You might think that I couldn't possibly have trouble fitting Pilates and cardio exercise into my schedule. After all, I exercise for a living, right?

Well, it's not that simple. Sure, when I film my television shows and videos, I am exercising. But I film only 3 months out of the year. The rest of the time my career involves sedentary tasks such as writing, planning, and talking on the phone. I have to make a concerted effort to fit exercise into my day, just like everyone else.

To better balance my life, I wrote down short-term and long-term goals for myself and established a vision of where I wanted to be. You can do the same. Write down three things you want to get out of your life and include your fitness goal, whether it's losing weight, getting back into shape after pregnancy, or strengthening a weak back. When you do that, you will see that doing Pilates and other exercise becomes a means to an end, helping you to make your workouts a priority in your life.

I also learned how to give myself a break. I try to realize that on some days certain things aren't going to get done. My family is priority number one, so at 3:00 P.M. every day, I put aside my work, forget about the dirty dishes in the sink, ignore the ringing telephone, and become 100 percent "mommy." I help my two daughters with their homework, shuttle them to tennis or lacrosse practice, and am completely present to listen, talk, and play.

The household chores will always be there, but my kids will even-

The Power of 10

There are so many days when I'm traveling or I simply can't fit in an entire routine. So I do what I can even if it is only a 5- or 10-minute workout. It's hard to believe that 10 minutes will do any good, but it does! Research from the University of Pittsburgh shows that people who exercise in 10-minute spurts may exercise more consistently overall than those who strive for 30 minutes.

tually grow up. Establishing those priorities helped me to carve out time for my girls, my husband, and myself.

I know that in order to be a good mom, I need to stay fit. Practicing Pilates regularly is one of the best ways to alleviate the pressures of daily life.

I try to exercise in the morning, before the day's activity begins, and do routines that are the most effective, such as the ones I've chosen for this section. For example, I wake up most mornings and do something cardio, such as a 20- to 30-minute walk/run. When I return or jump off the treadmill, I do my Pilates. I like the way the walk/run warms up my body. Breaking a little sweat helps me to feel more flexible during my Pilates session.

Whenever work and family responsibilities threaten to gobble up my exercise time, I remind myself that exercise is a proven way to reduce stress and anxiety—and it's a natural tranquilizer. Exercise also helps me to sleep better, which in turn gives me a much-needed good night's rest and allows me to wake up feeling refreshed. I feel that exercise is my mental filter, flushing out any grouchiness. It's only fair to me and my family that I stick to a regular fitness schedule. (For more on the benefits of including regular aerobic exercise in your routine, see part 4.)

Preplanning meals a week at a time also helps free up time to exercise during the day. It's easy to skip Pilates when you need to run a quick errand to the grocery store to pick up something for dinner. To avoid dinnertime chaos, I use Sunday as my meal-planning day. I prepare as much as I can for the week ahead. I pick out recipes for the week, make sure I have the ingredients on hand, and pre-chop much of the food. For example, I bake or broil chicken so that during the week I have chicken for salads or fajitas. (In part 4, you'll find specific advice on how to eat right and make healthy choices to supplement your exercise program.)

My 10-MINUTE Hip, Thigh, and Butt Routine

To perform better at gymnastics, I took years of ballet lessons, and you'll notice that a lot of the following exercises are balletlike. They're not traditional Pilates movements, but I've added a Pilates-esque twist to all of them. They all work the core abdominal muscles as well as target the muscles in your hips, inner thighs, outer thighs, fronts and backs of the thighs, and buttocks. As an added plus, by stretching your joints and muscles, they'll help you lengthen your legs, creating the long, lean, supple look of a dancer. I've also added some tried-and-true moves that, by working your gluteus maximus (the muscle that forms your buttocks), will help you make your backside your *best* side!

Make each exercise in the sequence last for about a minute. If the exercise requires you to repeat on the other side of your body, then do 30 seconds for each side. For most people, that means 10 to 20 repetitions, but go at your own pace. Move slowly and breathe throughout the movement. Aim to do each repetition the most effectively that you can. Remember, in every move, to focus on your center. Pull up through your pelvic muscles and press your belly button toward your spine.

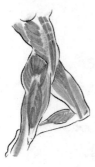

Ballet Brush Front

Benefits

A fantastic leg shaper, this works your inner and front thighs as well as warms up your leg muscles for the rest of the routine.

Pilates Pointer

▶ Begin moving from your abs first, then the top of your inner thigh, then the rest of your leg down to your toes.

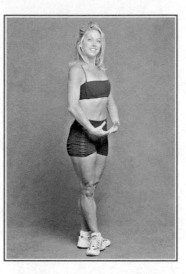

A. Begin in the fifth ballet position, with your hands in front of your waist, your navel pulled flat toward your spine, and your feet turned out with the heel of your right foot against the toe of your left.

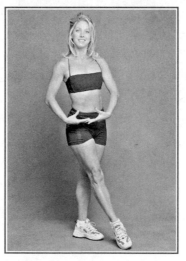

B. Use the strength in your abs to keep your balance as you inhale and slide your right big toe forward on a diagonal. Exhale as you return to the starting position. Repeat for 30 seconds, then switch legs.

Ballet Brush Side

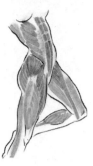

A. Begin in fifth position, with your hands in front of your waist, your navel pulled flat toward your spine, and your feet turned out with the heel of your right foot against the toe of your left.

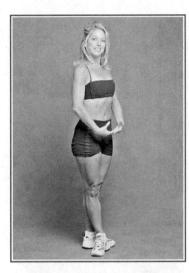

B. Use the strength in your abs to keep your balance as you inhale and put your body weight onto your left leg, bend your left knee, raise your arms to the sides, and slide your pointed right foot to the side. Try to do all of this in a fluid motion. Exhale as you return to the starting position. Repeat for 30 seconds, then switch legs.

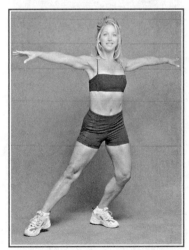

Benefits

This move works the entire thigh area, especially your inner and outer thighs.

Pilates Pointers

► Whenever you feel unbalanced, focus on your abs. Zip them up into that imaginary corset, and you'll regain your balance quickly.

► Feel your inner thighs connect to the lower region of your abs.

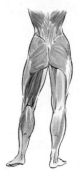

Plié

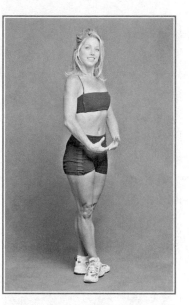

Benefits

Also borrowed from ballet, this move targets your entire lower body, especially your buttocks, inner thighs, and calves.

Pilates Pointers

► Press your heels together as you squat. This will help you stay balanced as well as keep your abs zipped up.

► Keep your back straight and your spine long. Think of good posture.

A. Begin in fifth position, with your hands in front of your waist, your abs pulled flat toward your spine, and your feet turned out with the heel of your right foot against the toe of your left.

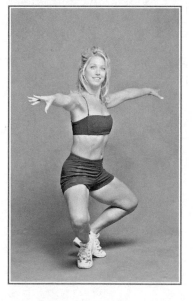

B. Use the strength in your abs to keep your balance as you inhale, bring your heels together, rise onto the balls of your feet, and squat down, bringing your knees to the sides. Extend your arms to the sides for balance. Exhale as you press through your inner thighs to rise. Repeat.

Relevé

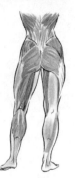

A. Stand with your weight on your right foot, your abs pressed flat against your spine, and your hands on your hips. Bend your left knee and raise your left foot behind your right calf, as shown.

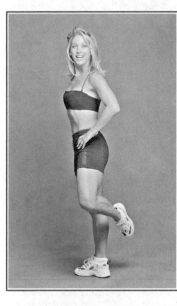

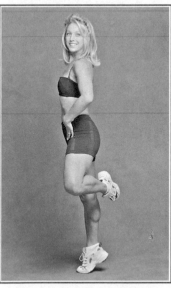

B. Using the strength of your abs to keep your balance, inhale and rise onto the ball of your right foot, as shown. Exhale as you lower. Repeat for 30 seconds, then switch legs.

Benefits

This move targets the backs of your legs and buttocks, plus your calves. You'll have shapely legs.

Pilates Pointers

► Try to maintain good posture, positioning your shoulders above your hips and your waist above your arches.

► If you feel off balance, use a chair for support, placing your hands on the back of the chair.

► Zip up your abs like a natural girdle.

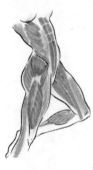

Leg Extension Sequence

Benefits

This targets your thighs and lengthens and strengthens your legs.

This is a great rehabilitation exercise for your knee. Conditioning the muscles surrounding your knee will help keep it healthy. It's also great for the lower region of your abs.

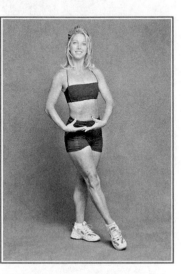

A. Begin with your hands in front of your waist, your abs engaged, and your right foot pointed slightly in front of your left. Inhale and use the strength in your abs to keep your balance as you slide your right big toe forward on a diagonal, as shown.

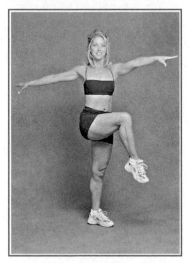

B. Using your abs to continue keeping your balance, exhale and raise your right knee, making sure to keep your hipbones level and your back flat. Extend your arms from your shoulders for balance and keep your shoulders relaxed.

"Make time for exercise—the earlier the better!"

Pilates Pointers

► Many people subconsciously turn one hipbone higher than the other during this exercise. To check your hips, periodically place an index finger on each hipbone to see if they are level.

► You'll feel this in your quadriceps (the muscles that form the front of your thighs).

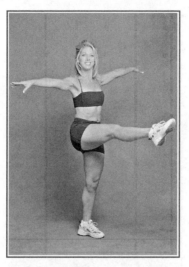

C. Keep your knee at hip level as you inhale and extend your right foot.

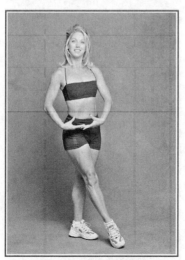

D. Exhale, bend your right knee, and return to the starting position. Repeat the sequence for 30 seconds, then switch legs.

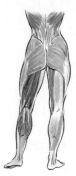

Benefits

This exercise is an excellent bun firmer and hip slimmer, which will reshape your bottom half.

Pilates Pointers

► It's easy to arch your back during this exercise. Keep it flat by pulling those abs up and in.

► Sit back; your weight should be through your heels.

Sitting Pose Sequence

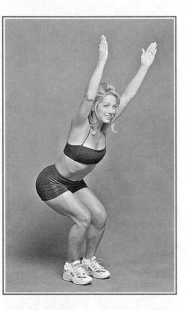

A. Stand with your feet slightly apart, your inner thighs raised, and your abs in and flat toward your spine. Keeping your back straight, inhale and sit back as though you were sitting into a chair. Simultaneously raise your arms overhead, as shown, making sure to keep your shoulders relaxed.

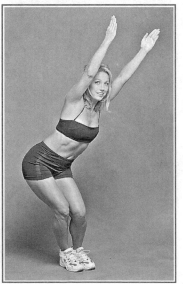

B. Exhale and extend through your fingertips to the left, bringing your entire torso in that direction, as shown. You should feel a stretch along your right side. Press through your right hip, starting to circle your hips back clockwise as you continue to circle your arms forward.

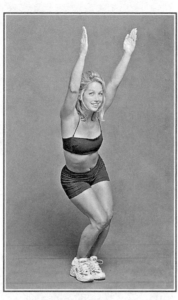

C. Inhale and continue to circle your arms toward the right as you circle your hips toward the left, making sure to keep your abs engaged.

D. Once you've made a complete revolution, bring your body back to center with your arms extended outward in front from your shoulders, as shown. Hold for 10 seconds, breathing normally. Then bring your arms back overhead and repeat the sequence in the opposite direction.

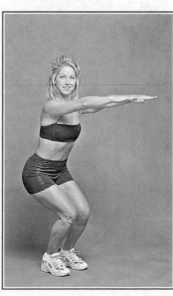

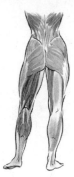

Bun Lifter

Benefit

Great for the glutes—the muscles that form your buttocks—this will help you look fantastic in jeans.

Pilates Pointer

▶ Keep your hipbones level. Imagine that you're balancing a ruler on your lower back. Don't let it slide off.

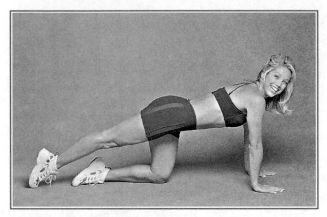

A. Get on all fours with your hands under your shoulders and your knees under your hips. Extend your right leg behind your body, with your toes on the floor, as shown.

B. Keep your abs pulled toward your spine as you inhale and raise your right heel and leg up, as shown, feeling the exercise in your buttocks. Exhale and lower. Repeat for 30 seconds, then switch legs.

Denise-eology . . .

"Imagine that your butt is a sponge, and you're squeezing out every last drop of water."

Bottom Firmer Sequence

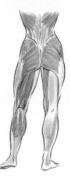

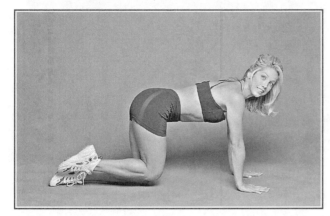

A. Still on all fours, as in the previous move, with your hands under your shoulders and your knees under your hips, lift your right knee from the floor, as shown.

Benefit
This move firms your entire buttock area.

Pilates Pointer
▶ When you bring one knee over to the other side, press into both palms equally to keep your torso properly aligned.

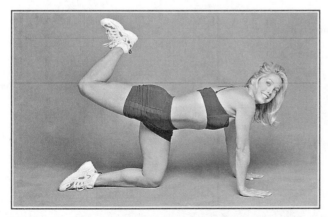

B. Pull your abs toward your spine as you inhale and bring your bent right leg up behind your body, pressing your right foot toward the ceiling.

—continued

Bottom Firmer Sequence

—continued

Denise-eology . . .

"Squeeze your buttocks anywhere, anytime—turn that idle time into exercise time."

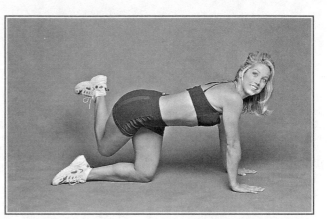

C. Exhale and bring your right knee toward the left, as shown, past the calf of your left leg. As you work through this exercise, you should feel it from your buttocks to your outer buttocks and outer thigh. Raise your right knee back up and repeat the sequence for 30 seconds before switching legs.

Leg Beats

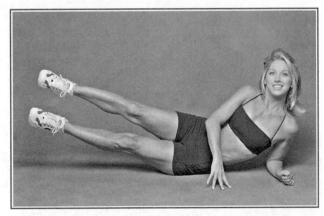

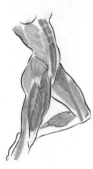

Lie on your left side with your legs extended and slightly in front of the plane of your body. Lean on your left forearm and place your right hand in front of you for balance. Inhale and use the strength of your abs to lift both legs up, as shown, feeling the exercise in your right buttock, hip, and thigh. Exhale and lower your bottom leg, then inhale and raise it. Repeat several times for 30 seconds. Then switch sides and repeat.

Benefits

This works your obliques (outer abs), buttocks, and inner thighs.

Pilates Pointers

► Make sure that your hips are stacked on top of each other; don't allow your right hipbone to collapse back.

► Feel your inner thighs connect to the lower region of your abs.

Denise-eology . . .

"I don't know anyone who doesn't want shapely legs. In just 10 minutes a day, you can tighten, tone, and shape your legs to achieve a great-looking lower body."

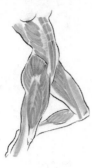

Inner Thigh Firmer

Benefit

Tones and strengthens your inner thighs.

Pilates Pointers

► Keep the movement slow and controlled. Allow the muscles in your abs and legs to do the work, not momentum.

► Feel your inner thighs and the lower region of your abs.

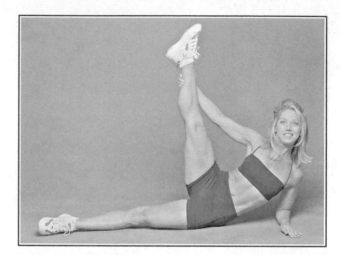

A. Lie on your left side with your left leg extended and your left forearm on the floor for balance. Raise your right leg up and hold on to it with your right hand at whatever level feels comfortable.

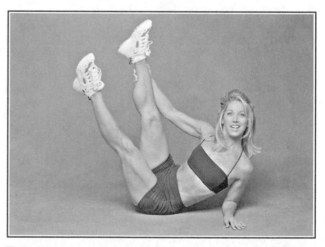

B. Engage your abs, navel in toward your spine, as you inhale and lift your left leg up, as shown, feeling the movement in your left inner thigh. Lower just a few inches and then raise again, pulsing your left leg up a few inches and down a few inches for 30 seconds as you exhale and inhale. Then switch sides and repeat.

My 5-MINUTE Resistance-Band Leg Workout

f you want to target those troublesome hips, butt muscles, and thighs but don't have the full 10 minutes for my previous routine, try this workout instead. It uses an elastic exercise band for added resistance, making each exercise a bit tougher.

Remember to maintain the Pilates emphasis during these moves: keep your abs engaged, your navel toward your spine, your shoulders relaxed, your chest open, and your spine long. As with the previous routine, spend 1 minute on each move. Believe me, after 5 minutes, you're going to feel as though you've gotten a great workout!

Denise-eology . . .

"Strong, well-toned muscles are the key to staying young."

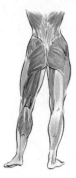

Hip and Outer Thigh Slimmer

Benefits

Besides specifically targeting the "saddlebag"-prone area, this move works your entire lower body, from your lower back to your abs to your thighs to your calves.

Pilates Pointer

► If you feel uncoordinated when first doing this move, go easy on yourself. Use a chair for balance or place one hand on a wall. Soon you'll be able to perform the exercise in a fluid, coordinated motion.

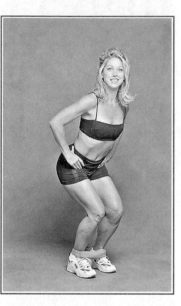

A. Stand with your hands on your hips and an exercise band around your ankles. Position your feet beneath your shoulders, stretching the band slightly. Bend your knees, inhale, and squat back, keeping your abs pressed against your spine, your back flat, and your chest open.

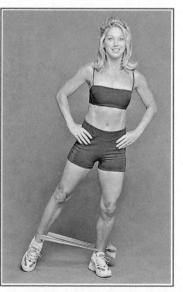

B. Exhale and press up into a standing position as you simultaneously extend your right leg to the right, feeling the effort in your outer right thigh, hip, and buttock. Return to the squat and repeat with the left leg. Continue squatting and alternating legs for 1 minute.

Buttocks Firmer

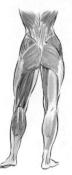

Stand with the exercise band around your ankles and your hands on your hips. Press your abs toward your spine and shift your body weight onto your left foot. Bring your right foot back behind you, as shown, feeling the motion in your buttocks. Bring your foot forward a bit and then back again, pulsing your leg forward a few inches and back a few inches for 30 seconds, as you breath normally. Then switch legs.

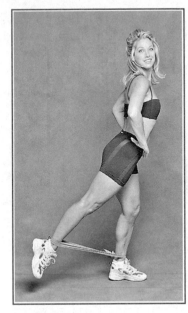

Benefit

Targets your buttock area, particularly the lower section that peeks out below your swimsuit.

Pilates Pointers

► Remember to pull in and up through your abs. Zip them up!

► If you're off balance, place your hands on a chair or on a wall for balance.

Denise-eology . . .

"Do these routines anytime, anywhere. Remember, your muscles don't know if you're on the bedroom floor or at a fancy gym."

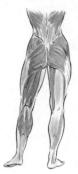

Hamstring Curl

Benefit

Firms and tones the backs of your thighs.

Pilates Pointers

► Remember to lengthen through your body before you lift your heel. Let an imaginary string pull the crown of your head toward the ceiling.

► Zip up your abs like an imaginary corset.

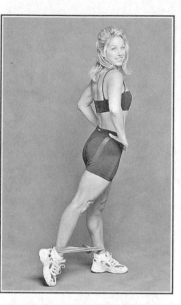

A. Stand with your hands on your hips and an exercise band around your ankles. Flatten your navel in toward your spine and bring your right lower leg back behind the plane of your body.

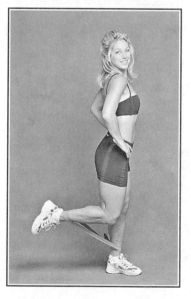

B. With your abs still engaged, exhale and curl your right heel up toward your buttocks, stopping when your right calf is parallel to the floor, as shown. Lower as you inhale. Repeat for 30 seconds, then switch legs.

Quad Firmer

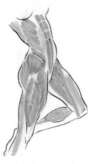

A. Stand with an exercise band around your ankles, your hands on your hips, and your navel in toward your spine. Put your body weight onto your left foot and bend your right knee, bringing the ball of your right foot onto the floor.

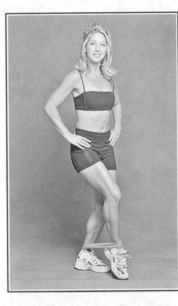

Benefits

This strengthens the fronts of your thighs and tones and firms your thighs, especially above the knee.

Pilates Pointer

► Create as much length as possible as you extend your leg from your hip joint all the way to your big toe.

B. Exhale and extend through your right toes, straightening your leg by moving only your lower leg, as shown. Bend your knee back to the starting position as you inhale. Repeat for 30 seconds, then switch legs.

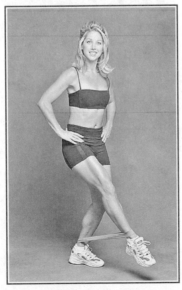

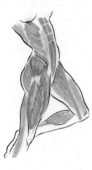

Inner Thigh Shaper

Benefit

This tones your inner thighs, preventing them from rubbing together or jiggling when you walk.

Pilates Pointer

► Keep your hips level throughout this exercise. Press an index finger against each hipbone periodically so you can easily check your posture.

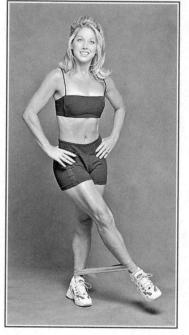

Stand with an exercise band around your ankles, your hands on your hips, and your abs engaged. Put your body weight onto your left foot. Straighten your right leg in front so that the right ball of your foot is on the floor. Exhale and sweep your right foot toward the left, as shown, in front of your left leg. You should feel the effort in your right inner thigh. Inhale as you return to the starting position. Repeat for 30 seconds, then switch legs.

Denise-eology . . .

"Don't be your own worst critic.
Wipe away those negative thoughts.
Be kind to yourself and
do something positive."

My 10-MINUTE Upper Body Routine

A strong, firm, flexible upper body will improve your posture, make your lower body appear slimmer, and help you more easily accomplish everyday tasks such as carrying groceries.

Important muscles in your upper back and along your spine help keep you upright. This routine will tone those muscles. It will also help firm the area along the back of your upper arms, a common trouble spot in women, as well as help create a long, sleek-looking back, perfect to show off in a backless dress. For men, this routine will help build an upper body, shaping your arms, chest, and shoulders.

The following series of poses incorporate a Pilates emphasis. Keep the powerhouse—your center—strong. Keep your abs pulled up and in toward your spine for every single one of them. They'll help you strengthen and sculpt all of the muscles in your upper body—your chest, shoulders, upper back, and arms.

Do this routine at least twice a week, as a complement to the Pilates programs in part 2 of this book.

The first time you complete this sequence, do it without weights.

After that, try a set of light dumbbells. If you're just starting out, begin with 2- to 3-pound weights in each hand. Then work up in 2- to 5-pound increments as you feel stronger.

I use 8-pound weights for most of the exercises. If you've been working out for a while, you might be able to start with 8s. If you're a guy, you can probably start with 10-pound weights and work up. My husband does this routine with 15- to 20-pound weights.

I recommend this rule of thumb for choosing weights: When you are doing 12 repetitions of an exercise, the final 2 repetitions should feel tough. If they don't, the weight is too light, and you should challenge yourself by adding a couple of pounds. If you start to struggle long before the 10th repetition, the weight is too heavy.

Also, you want to maintain good form. If you find the exercise tough to execute properly, the weight is probably too heavy.

Because some muscles, such as those in your shoulders, are stronger than others, such as your triceps (along the back of your upper arms), you may find that you must adjust the amount of weight you lift for different exercises. Remember, your body will tell you what you can lift. If you feel wobbly and unsteady during the movement, the weight is too heavy. Lift the weight slowly and fluidly.

Make each exercise in the sequence last for about a minute. If the exercise requires you to repeat on the other side of your body, then do 30 seconds for each side. For most people, that means 10 to 20 repetitions, but go at your own pace. Move slowly and breathe throughout the movement.

Denise-eology . . .

"A little muscle looks marvelous—and works miracles for your metabolism."

Zip-Up
(Upright Row)

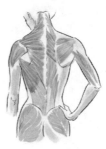

A. Stand with your knees slightly bent and your abs pressed up and in toward your spine. Hold a pair of dumbbells in front of you slightly lower than waist level with the ends of the dumbbells touching.

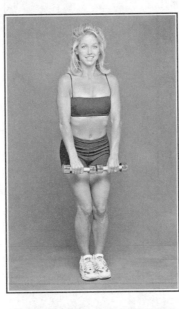

Benefits

This exercise tones your upper back and shoulders.

Pilates Pointers

► Feel as though you are zipping up as you engage your abs in your center. As your hands rise along the center of your body, imagine that they are zipping up a corset, pulling everything in.

► Retract your shoulder blades downward. Don't hunch your shoulders upward.

B. Keep the dumbbells pressed together as you inhale and raise your hands up, bringing your elbows to the sides. Stop once your hands reach chest level. Exhale as you lower them. Repeat.

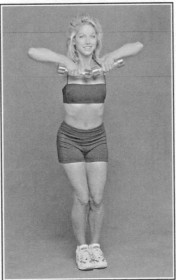

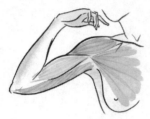

Strong Man

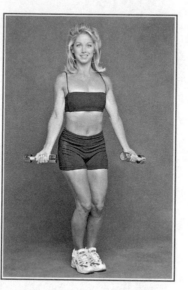

Benefit

Tones and strengthens your biceps, the muscles along the front of your upper arms.

Pilates Pointers

► Keep your elbows pressed in toward your sides throughout the move. The area of your arm from your shoulders to your elbows should remain motionless.

► Position your knees over your shoelaces.

A. Stand with your knees slightly bent and your abs engaged, navel in toward your spine. Hold a pair of dumbbells at your sides, with your palms facing up.

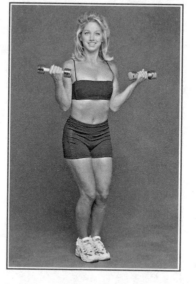

B. Inhale as you curl your hands toward your shoulders. Exhale as you lower them. Repeat.

Side Raise

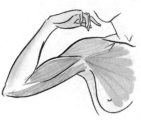

A. Stand with your knees slightly bent and your abs engaged, navel in toward your spine. Holding a pair of dumbbells in front of you slightly lower than waist level and with your palms facing each other, bend forward slightly from your waist.

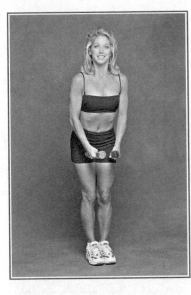

Benefit

Tones your shoulders, specifically your medial (middle) deltoids.

Pilates Pointers

► Keep the movement slow and controlled. Don't jerk your arms out to the sides.

► Focus on the core, keeping your abs strong.

B. Keep your shoulders low as you exhale and raise your arms to the sides. Stop once your hands reach shoulder level. Inhale as you lower your arms. Repeat.

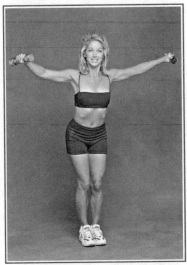

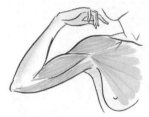

Alternating Arms

Benefit

This exercise tones your shoulders, specifically your anterior (front) deltoids.

Pilates Pointers

► Keep your neck long and shoulders low. Create as much space between your shoulders and your ears as you can.

► Slower is better. Use smooth, flowing movements.

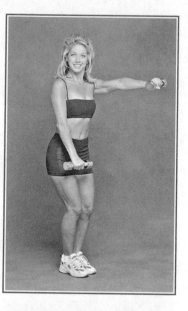

A. Stand with your knees slightly bent and your abs engaged, navel in toward your spine. Hold a pair of dumbbells at your sides, with your palms facing behind you. While keeping your shoulders low, exhale and raise your left arm up in front of your body, as shown, bringing your hand to chest level while keeping the arm extended with a slight bend of the elbow.

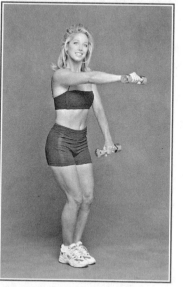

B. Inhale as you lower your arm. Repeat with your right arm, as shown, and continue switching for 1 minute.

Ladybug

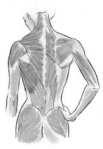

A. Stand with your knees slightly bent and your abs engaged, navel in toward your spine. Holding a pair of dumbbells below your chest with your elbows bent and palms facing each other, bend forward from your waist at about a 45-degree angle.

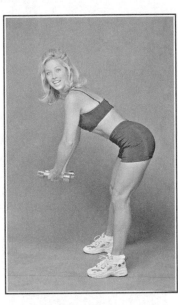

Benefit

Tones and strengthens your upper back.

Pilates Pointers

► Keep your back flat throughout the move. Try not to curl your spine in either direction.

► Lead with your elbows.

► Don't scrunch your neck or shoulders.

► Keep your abs strong to support your back.

B. Inhale and raise both dumbbells up to shoulder level, keeping your elbows bent throughout the movement. Exhale as you lower the dumbbells. Repeat.

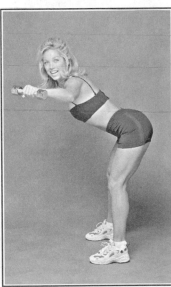

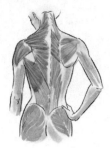

Arm Extension

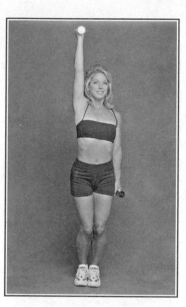

Benefit

Tones your arms, especially the triceps, the muscles along the back of your upper arms.

Pilates Pointers

► Use a lighter weight for this exercise.

► Allow the hand of your raised arm to move slightly away from your head, with your thumb pointed out. This will further target that triceps area.

► Take your time and control the movement.

► Focus on your center, the core of your body.

A. Stand with your knees slightly bent and your abs engaged, navel in toward your spine. Hold a pair of dumbbells at your sides, with your palms facing your thighs. Exhale and raise your right arm in front of you and overhead, extending it toward the ceiling, as shown. Extend your left arm toward the floor.

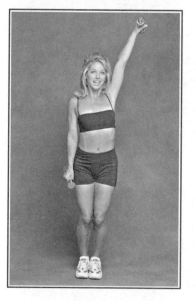

B. Inhale as you switch arms, bringing your left arm up and your right arm down. Continue switching for 1 minute.

Triceps Toner

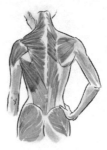

A. Stand with your knees slightly bent and your abs engaged, navel in toward your spine. Holding a dumbbell in your right hand, extend your right arm toward the ceiling. Use your left hand to support your right arm, as shown.

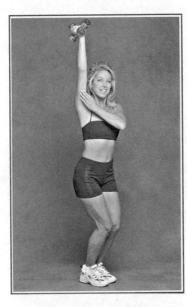

B. As you inhale, bend your right elbow, bringing the dumbbell behind your head, as shown. Then exhale and press the dumbbell up to the starting position. Repeat for 30 seconds, then switch arms.

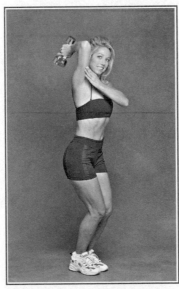

Benefit

This exercise further tones your triceps muscles, eliminating underarm flab.

Pilates Pointers

► Keep the top of your arm— from your shoulder to your elbow—motionless.

► Feel your triceps muscle working.

► Try not to arch your back.

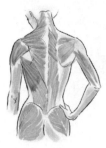

Double-Arm Row

Benefits

This move improves your posture by strengthening all the muscles along your spine and upper back.

Pilates Pointers

► As you press back with your elbows, focus on the area between your shoulder blades. Use that area to pull the weights in toward your torso.

► Keep your chest open, but your ribs down.

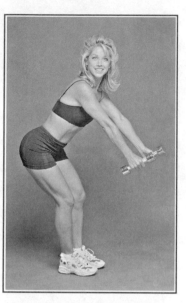

A. Stand with your knees slightly bent and your abs engaged, navel in toward your spine. Hinge at your waist. Holding a dumbbell in each hand with your palms facing one another, extend your arms so that your hands are on the same plane as your shoulders. (If you were standing straight up, they'd be parallel with the floor).

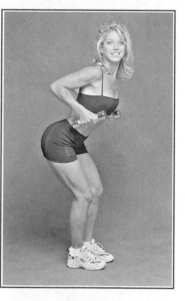

B. Keep your shoulders pulled down and away from your ears as you exhale and bring your elbows back behind your body. Inhale and return to the starting position. Repeat.

Denise-eology . . .
"I sometimes do arm exercises when I watch the news on TV. Do them whenever you have time.**"**

Overhead Press

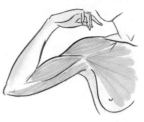

A. Stand in a lunge position, with your right leg extended behind your body and your left leg in front, bent. Pull your navel in toward your spine. Bend your arms and bring the dumbbells to shoulder level with your palms facing forward.

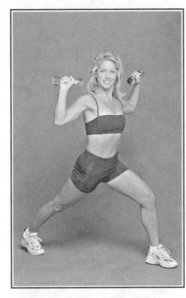

Benefit

This move tones your shoulder muscles, giving a beautiful shape to your upper body.

Pilates Pointers

► Imagine that you're Atlas, holding the world above your head. Your entire body needs to be strong and stable throughout this exercise.

► Focus on keeping your "core" engaged as you press up, and don't let your back arch.

B. Keeping your abs engaged and your shoulders down and away from your ears, exhale and press the dumbbells up, extending your arms. Inhale as you lower your arms. Repeat.

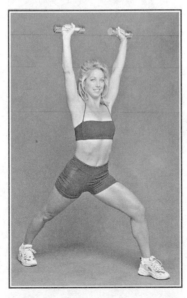

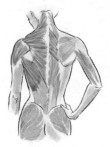

Rotator Strengthener

Benefits

This exercise strengthens the small rotator cuff muscles in your shoulders. These are the muscles that tend to wear and tear with age, preventing you from doing something as simple as raising your arms overhead.

Pilates Pointers

► This is a very small movement but very effective.

► I do this exercise with a weighted ball, but you can also do it with dumbbells or no resistance at all.

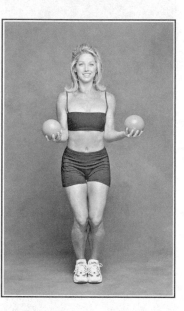

A. Stand with your knees slightly bent and your abs engaged, navel in toward your spine. Palm a weighted medicine ball in each hand, or grasp a pair of dumbbells. Bend your elbows and bring them next to your ribs with your palms facing up.

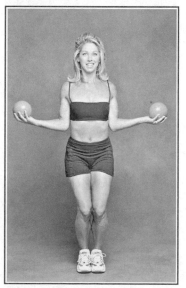

B. Keeping your elbows against your ribs, exhale and rotate your forearms out to the sides, then inhale and rotate them back to the starting position. Repeat.

My 10-MINUTE Advanced Abdominal Routine

Pilates targets your abs in ways that no other form of exercise does. This mini-routine contains some of the toughest Pilates moves. Use it when you're short on time, when you're feeling up for a challenge, or when you want to "change it up" a bit.

The routine works all the areas of the abdominal region as well as the back. Each exercise is specific and will target your rectus abdominis, your obliques, your transverse abdominis, as well as your back—muscles that work together to function like a girdle for your entire torso.

Remember, keeping your abs engaged and navel in toward your spine gives you control of all of these movements. Because some of these movements are very challenging, this is a good routine in which to try my percussion breathing technique described on page 33.

Make each exercise in the sequence last for about a minute. If the exercise requires you to repeat on the other side of your body, then do 30 seconds for each side. For most people, that means 10 to 20 repetitions.

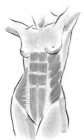

Benefits

This tightens your lower belly and pelvic area, giving more support to your lower back.

Pilates Pointer

► Keep your elbows out to the sides as you do this move. (You shouldn't be able to see your elbows.) This will prevent you from using your hands to lift your head. Instead, relax your head into your fingertips.

The Frog

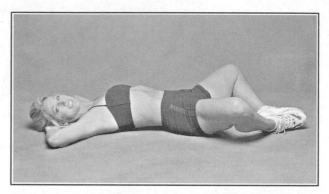

A. Lie on your back with your knees bent and to the sides and with the bottoms of your feet touching. Rest your head back into your fingertips, keeping your elbows out to the sides.

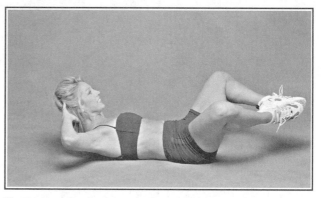

B. Exhale as you pull your abs toward your spine and curl your hipbones and ribs toward one another, raising both feet and shoulders off the floor. Inhale as you lower. Repeat.

Double-Leg Lift

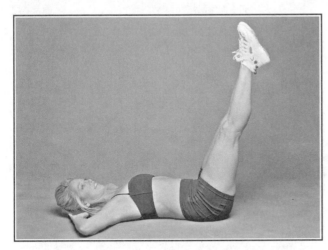

A. Lie on your back with your head resting back into your fingertips, your elbows out to the sides, and your legs extended in the air, forming a 90-degree angle with your torso.

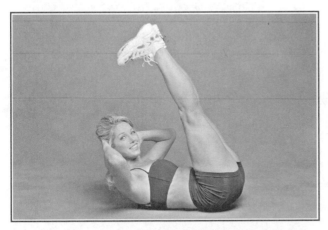

B. Flatten your navel in toward your spine, engage your abs, and exhale as you curl your hipbones toward your ribs, raising your feet and shoulders. Inhale as you lower. Repeat.

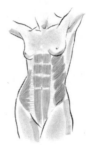

Benefit

This strengthens your entire rectus abdominis muscle, running from your sternum (breastbone) to your pelvic bone.

Pilates Pointers

► To resist the tendency to cheat and use momentum, focus on the area below your navel. Curl up by pressing that area in and up. Also keep it flat as you lower your legs.

► Pull your navel in, anchor your torso, and squeeze your inner thighs together.

Corkscrew

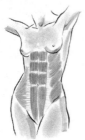

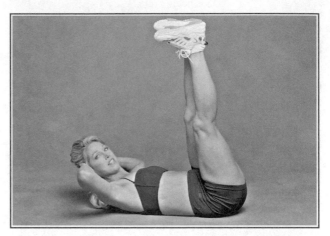

Benefit

This move strengthens the sides of your abdominal area, helping you to shrink your waist.

Pilates Pointers

► Start with a small circle. As you gain strength and coordination, you'll be able to make larger and larger circles.

► Feel as though your torso is anchored to the floor.

► Keep the abs in total control of this movement.

Lie on your back with your head resting back into your fingertips and your elbows out to the sides. Extend your legs in the air, forming a 90-degree angle with your torso. Engage your abs, flatten your navel in toward your spine as you inhale and lower your legs to the right, as shown, keeping your feet and knees pressed together. Continue in a circle to the right, then down, then to the left—exhaling when needed—and keeping your knees and feet together as you bring your feet slightly to the left and back up to the start. Circle to the right for 30 seconds and then reverse direction.

Denise-eology . . .
"Respect your body.
God gave us each
one body. Say yes to life!"

Can-Can

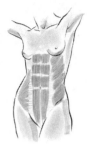

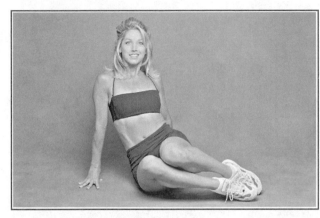

A. Sit with your weight on your "sit bones," your hands on the floor behind you for balance, your knees bent, and your toes touching the floor. Keep your ankles and knees pressed together as you inhale and lower your knees to the right, as shown.

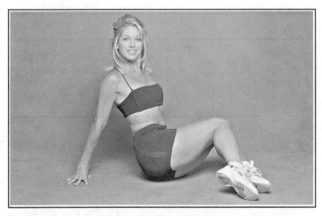

B. Exhale and use your belly to pull your legs back up. Inhale and then exhale as you lower them to the left, as shown. Repeat from side to side for 1 minute.

Benefits

This move focuses on your obliques (the muscles that form your waist) as well as massages and releases tightness in your lower back.

Pilates Pointers

► Don't allow your knees to simply fall to the side. Use your abs to slowly lower them. Make every part of the exercise count.

► The key is to stabilize your abs. Work from the inside out.

Can-Can
Extension—more challenging

Pilates Pointers

► Try not to lean back as you extend your legs. Use the strength in your abs to keep your torso stable.

► Squeeze your inner thighs.

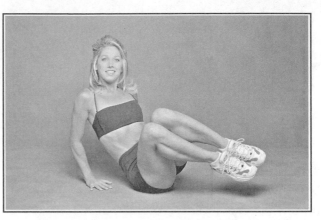

A. Sit with your weight on your sit bones, your hands on the floor behind you for balance, your knees bent, and your toes touching the floor. Keep your ankles and knees pressed together as you inhale and lower your knees to the right, as shown.

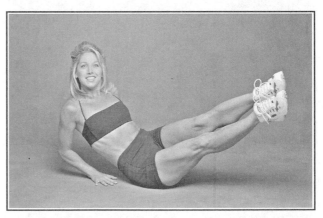

B. Pull your navel in toward your spine and raise your feet into the air, extending your legs as you exhale, as shown. Inhale as you bend your knees, bring them to the left, and then exhale as you extend your feet. Continue repeating the sequence.

Plank

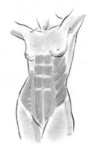

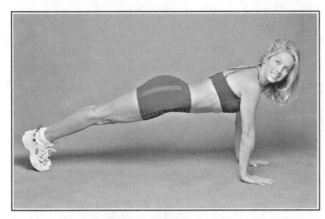

A. Get in the basic plank position, with your hands under your shoulders and weight on the balls of your feet. Pull your navel in toward your spine and try to lengthen your body from your head to your feet. Adjust your feet if needed.

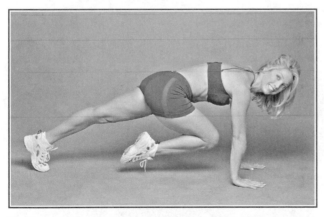

B. Keeping your abs strong, exhale and slowly bring your right knee in toward your left shoulder.

Benefits

This works your entire abdominal area as well as your sides and back.

Pilates Pointers

► Make sure that your hips stay parallel to the floor. Use the strength of your abs to keep your torso stable, not tipped to one side.

► Try to imagine balancing a glass of water on your back.

► Focus on the lower region of your abs.

—continued

Plank
—continued

Denise-eology . . .

"To prevent belly
bloating, don't
chew gum, don't
sip from a straw,
don't drink too many
carbonated beverages,
and eat slowly."

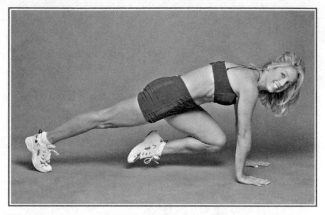

C. Inhale, return your right leg to the starting position, and then exhale and bring your left knee in toward your right shoulder, as shown. Repeat the entire sequence alternating legs for 1 minute. Take a rest when needed.

Low Hover

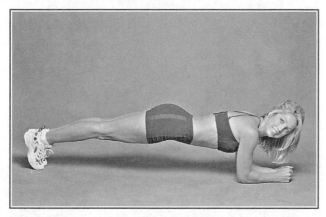

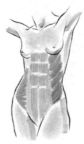

Lie on your belly. Place your elbows on the floor next to your shoulders and hold your hands together, so that your arms form a triangle. Pull in and up through your abs, flattening them toward your spine. Focusing on your abs, inhale and rise into the hover position, as shown. Hold the pose as you exhale and inhale three times. Then lower, rest, and repeat.

Benefit

This exercise works your entire abdominal area with special focus on the transverse abdominis.

Pilates Pointer

► Though your upper body must make some effort to support the weight of your body, your abs should be doing most of the work. Your abs are the focus. They are fighting gravity.

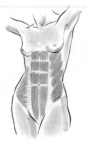

Oblique Strengthener

Benefits

This move, which improves your balance, strengthens your arms and shoulders while stretching and strengthening your waist and hips. It's also my husband's favorite—it targets those "love handles" that we all don't like. It worked great for him.

Pilates Pointers

► Challenge yourself to keep your hipbones stacked on top of each other. To do so, use those outer abs to keep your torso perpendicular to the floor.

► This is very advanced but very effective, so you only have to do three on each side.

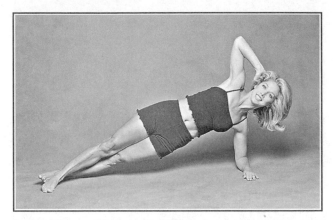

A. Sit with your left hip on the floor and your legs extended. Bring your right arm behind your head. With your left forearm on the floor, inhale and use your abs to lift into position, as shown, balancing on the outer edge of your left foot and left forearm.

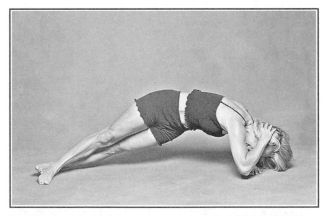

B. Exhale and slowly lower your right elbow toward the floor. Use your abs to rise to the starting position. Repeat three times, then switch sides.

Double-Leg Tummy Tuck

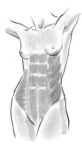

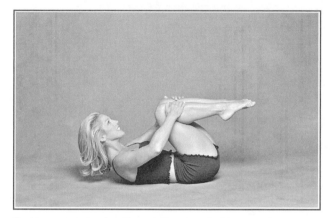

A. Lie on your back with your knees pulled in toward your chest. Rest your hands just below your knees and inhale as you use your abs to raise your shoulders off the floor, as shown.

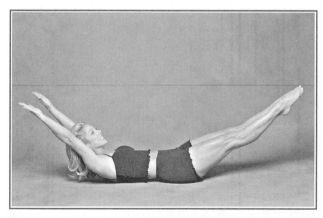

B. Exhale as you press your arms and legs out, making sure to engage and move from your abs. Extend through your fingertips and toes. Hold and then inhale as you bring your knees in toward your chest when you need to rest. Repeat three to six times.

Benefits

This move works your abs 100 percent and will teach you how to keep your abs contracted and stabilized. It will also teach you to coordinate your breathing with arm and leg movements. It also stretches your arms and legs.

Pilates Pointers

► Really create length in your body by elongating through your fingertips and toes. And be sure to keep those shoulders away from your ears.

► Make sure your lower back stays on the floor while you extend your legs outward but in control.

► Anchor your torso to the floor.

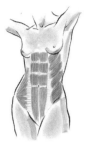

Benefit

This is a great finishing move because it requires quite a bit of lower abdominal strength to achieve liftoff.

Pilates Pointer

► At first your hips and feet may not leave the floor. Keep trying. Eventually, they'll be airborne!

Ab Lift

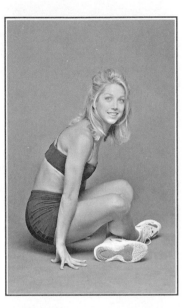

A. Sit on the floor with your legs crossed. Place your palms on the floor beside your hips.

B. Engage your abs and draw your navel in toward your spine as you inhale and sink your body weight onto your palms. Using your abs, raise your torso up, as shown, bringing your hips, buttocks, legs, and feet off the floor. Hold for as long as you can, exhaling and inhaling, using percussion breathing if needed. Lower, and then repeat three times.

Denise's Favorite Back Strengthener (The Swan)

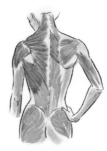

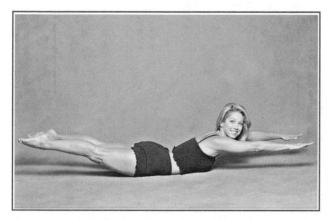

Lie on your belly, with your arms extended in front of you and your legs extended behind. Scoop your abs up against your spine so that your pubic bone presses into the floor. Inhale and lengthen through your legs and arms by pressing through your toes and fingers as you raise your heels and shoulders, as shown. Exhale and inhale normally, holding the pose for 10 seconds. Relax and repeat twice.

Benefits

Strengthens and stretches your abs, strengthens your entire back, and elongates your spine.

Pilates Pointers

► To keep those abs pulled in and up, imagine trying to lift your abdomen off the floor so that only your ribs and pubic bone touch the ground.

► Don't arch your back too much—think of your spine as long and lengthened.

Denise-eology . . .

"When you laugh,
    you're toning your tummy!
Laugh hard and laugh often."

My 10-MINUTE Healthy Back Routine

Too many people experience unnecessary back pain, and the consequences can be debilitating. That's why I recommend this routine to everyone—not just those who already have back problems—as a preventive program.

Most of us will feel back pain at some point during our lifetimes because we typically spend large portions of our days sitting. Even if you sit with perfect posture, the very nature of sitting shortens muscles that connect the tops of your legs to your hips. This pulls your pelvis forward, which in turn brings your spine into an undesirable alignment. Pregnancy can pull your pelvis even more, which is one reason that many pregnant women experience back pain.

This poor alignment brings the individual vertebra, joints, and disks that form your spine closer together, giving them less room and sometimes creating friction. It also stresses the muscles of your back and weakens the muscles of your abdomen. This in itself can inflict back pain. Also, because the muscles in your abs and back act as pillars that support your spine, weak and tight abdominal and back muscles can pull your spine further out of alignment.

The following routine reverses that process. It will help ensure that when you reach for something or try to pick something up, your back won't go out on you. These exercises will move your spine slowly and effectively in all directions—forward, back, to the sides, and in a twisting motion—keeping it supple, flexible, and healthy and creating more space between the disks, joints, and bones in your spine. This routine also improves the strength of the back extensor muscles that support your spine as well as your abdominals, helping you to stand with better posture automatically. Strong abdominals help take the pressure off your lower back muscles. They also help to bring your pelvis into the correct position.

Because these exercises work the back and abdominal muscles in concert, it's also a great postpregnancy routine to help you strengthen the muscle tone that you lost when your baby stretched out that tummy! You'll start noticing improvement within 3 weeks.

I have suggested this routine to many of my family and friends who complained to me about back pain. Every single one of them is now committed to the routine—and pain-free. If you have been diagnosed with a spinal concern, however—including disk degeneration, spinal stenosis, and disk herniation—please check with your doctor before attempting this program.

Make each exercise in the sequence last for about a minute. If the exercise requires you to repeat on the other side of your body, then do 30 seconds for each side. For most people, that means 10 to 20 repetitions.

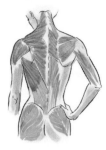

Neck-Shoulder-Back Relaxer

Benefits

As the name suggests, this move will release tension from your neck, shoulders, and back, readying you for the rest of the routine. Plus, it instantly relieves neck tension.

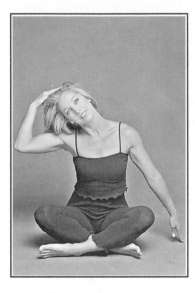

A. Sit comfortably with your legs crossed in front of you. Bring your body weight back onto your "sit bones," engage your abs, and lengthen through the crown of your head, as if a string were pulling your head up. Place your left hand on the floor. Exhale and lower your right ear toward your right shoulder, as shown. Gently use your right fingers to increase the stretch in your neck, holding for 20 seconds, taking deep, cleansing breaths.

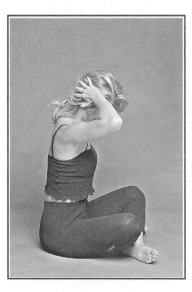

B. Inhale and roll your head forward, bringing your chin close to your upper chest. Gently use the fingers of both hands to increase the stretch to the back of your neck and shoulders, holding for 20 seconds, taking deep, cleansing breaths.

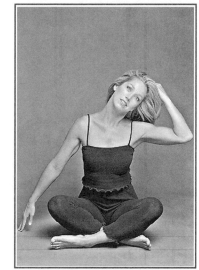

C. Exhale and roll your head to the left. Place your right hand on the floor. Gently use the fingers of your left hand to increase the stretch to the side of your neck as you hold for 20 seconds taking deep, cleansing breaths.

Pilates Pointers

► When you use your fingers to increase the stretch, don't jerk your head. Only lay your fingers against your head and allow gravity to pull your head over slightly.

► Retract your shoulders. Keep them down and back— not hunched.

► Elongate your neck.

Denise-eology . . .

"You are only as young as your spine."

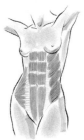

Lower Abdominal Strengthener with Towel

Benefit

This targets the lower region of your abs, the exact spot that gets weakened during pregnancy.

Pilates Pointer

► As you do the move, press your legs into the towel. That will automatically help you target your abs even more, because your top inner thighs are connected to your lower ab region.

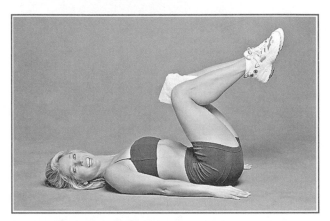

A. Lie with your back on the floor, your hands down at your sides, and a towel clenched between your knees. Lengthen your body from the crown of your head to your tailbone.

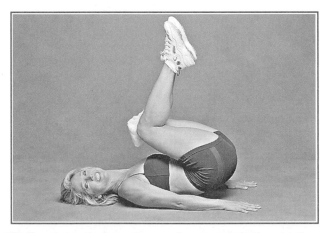

B. Press your abs toward your spine as you exhale and curl your hipbones toward your ribs. Inhale as you lower. Repeat.

Oblique Strengthener with Towel

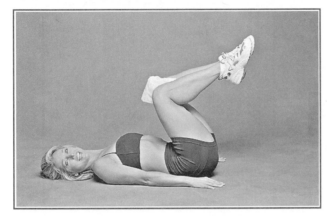

A. Lie with your back on the floor, your hands down at your sides, and a towel clenched between your knees. Lengthen your body from the crown of your head to your tailbone.

Benefit

Works your oblique muscles, which help your back muscles support your trunk and spine.

Pilates Pointers

► Your abs must stay strong and engaged.

► Keep your knees pressed into the towel as you lower to each side.

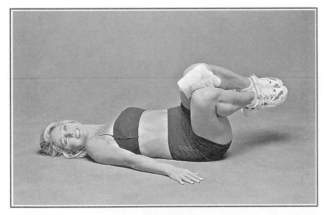

B. Engage your abs, navel in toward your spine, as you inhale and lower your knees slightly to the right.

—continued

Oblique Strengthener
with Towel

—continued

Denise-eology . . .

"Your spine is
your lifeline.
Keep it healthy
and strong!"

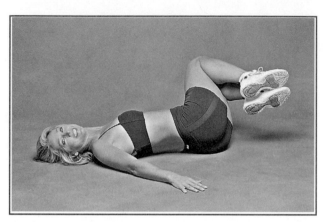

C. Exhale and use your abs to raise your knees to center, and then inhale as you lower them to the left, as shown. Repeat the sequence slowly and gently.

Bridge with Towel

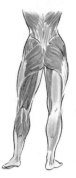

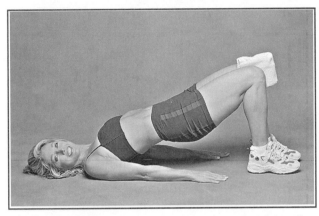

Lie on your back with your knees bent and your feet flat on the floor. Rest your arms at your sides, with your palms down and at about hip level. Squeeze a towel between your knees. Take a deep breath. Exhale as you contract your abs and curl your hips up, as shown, using your abs (not your buttocks or back) to lift your torso. You can use your hands for balance, but don't use them to push yourself up. Hold the position for 10 seconds. Relax and repeat twice.

Benefits

This move teaches you to use your abs to protect your back when it's in an arched position. It also stretches the hip flexors, strengthens the hamstrings along the back of the thighs, and tones your inner thighs. No more jiggles.

Pilates Pointers

► Try to keep your knees pressed into the towel so that you target your inner thighs and pelvic floor muscles.

► Try to lengthen your neck and relax your face muscles.

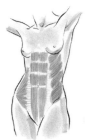

Perfect Ab Curl

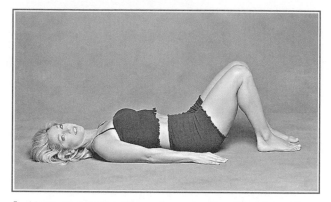

A. Lie on your back with your knees bent and feet flat on the floor. Extend your arms so that your hands rest on either side of your buttocks.

Benefits

This move strengthens the upper and lower region of your abs as well as increases the flexibility among the individual vertebra in your spine.

Pilates Pointers

► Relax your neck muscles and focus your eyes on your knees as you curl up.

► Scoop and hollow your abs.

► Try to touch your fingertips to your knees.

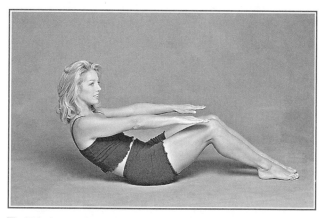

B. Exhale as you contract your abs and squeeze your inner thighs together to lift your shoulders up, bringing your ribs closer to your hips. Lift up until your shoulder blades are off the floor. Inhale as you release your shoulders slowly to the floor. Repeat.

Cat Stretch

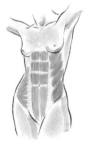

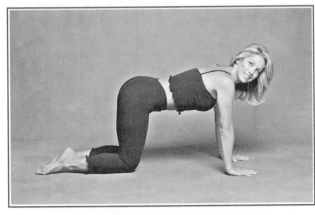

A. Get on all fours with your hands under your shoulders and knees under your hips. Press your navel in toward your spine.

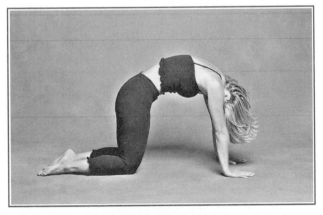

B. Exhale as you pull your abs up and in toward your spine even more, curling your hipbones down and forming a C shape with your spine. Scoop and hollow the abs.

Benefits

This pose stretches your back and strengthens your abs. It's one of the best exercises for your entire torso—front and back.

Pilates Pointers

► This is a great stretch to do first thing in the morning, even every day if you can.

► Keep your abs engaged as you round your back.

—continued

Cat Stretch
—continued

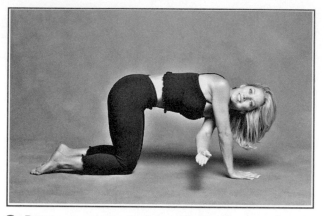

C. Return your spine to the flat position. Inhale as you thread your extended left arm under your body to the right, as shown, feeling a nice stretch along the left side of your back. Return your left hand to the floor and repeat with your right arm. Repeat the sequence.

Lower Back Strengthener

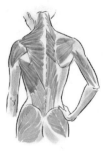

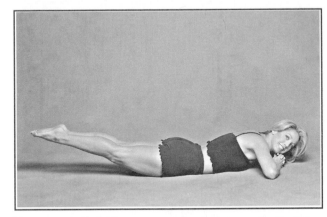

Lie on your belly, fold your arms in front of you, and rest your head into your folded arms. Scoop your abs against your spine so that your pubic bone presses into the floor. Lengthen your legs by pressing through your toes as you inhale and raise your heels up, as shown. Hold for about 3 to 6 seconds, lower, and repeat twice more.

Benefits

This move strengthens and stretches your abs, strengthens your lower back, and elongates your lower spine.

Pilates Pointers

► If you feel any pinching in your lower back, your abs are not engaged and navel not firmly in against your spine.

► Don't lift your legs too high; keep your spine long.

Denise-eology . . .

"We are reawakening thousands of muscle cells, we are increasing our energy and vitality, and best of all we are elevating our spirits."

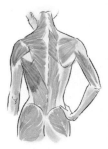

Benefit

This move strengthens the muscles of your middle and upper back.

Pilates Pointer

► To gain more lift in your upper torso, press your hands back toward your feet, keeping your abs strong the entire time.

Middle and Upper Back Strengthener

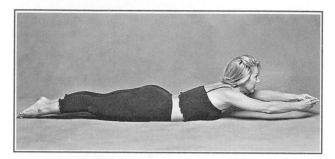

A. Lie on your belly with your legs extended behind you and your arms extended in front. Lift your abs toward your spine, and slightly squeeze your buttocks. Extend through your fingertips and toes, inhale, and bring your shoulders up, as shown.

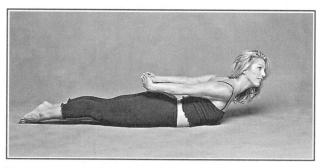

B. Keep your shoulders in position as you bring your arms back behind you, touching your fingertips. Hold for a second. Then relax and repeat twice.

Hamstring and Back Stretch Sequence

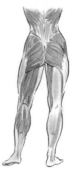

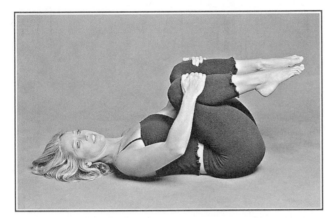

A. Lie on your back with your knees pulled in toward your chest and your hands resting just below your knees. Press your belly button toward your spine.

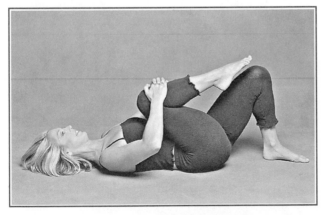

B. Lower your left foot to the floor. Bring your right knee in toward your chest, as shown, feeling a stretch along the back of your right leg and buttock.

Benefits

This relaxes your back after working it, positioning your spine in an opposite way from the lower and middle back strengtheners. This also stretches your hamstrings. Tight hamstrings often lead to a sore back by tugging your pelvis in the wrong direction, putting pressure on your lower back. So keep your hamstrings limber.

Pilates Pointers

► Lengthen your neck and relax your face muscles.

► Ease into this stretch and increase your range of movement.

—continued

Hamstring and Back Stretch Sequence

—continued

Pilates Pointer

► Straighten your leg during the final hamstring stretch *only* if you can keep your lower back from arching.

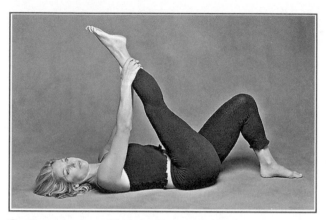

C. Straighten your right leg and use your hands on your calf to gently increase the stretch, breathing deeply.

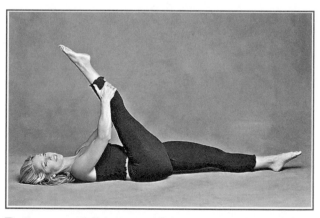

D. If you can, straighten your left leg against the floor. Hold for 20 to 30 seconds and then repeat the sequence on the other side.

Spinal Twist and Trunk Rotation

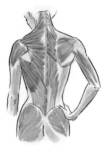

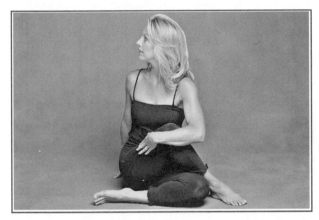

A. Sit with your legs extended to front. Bend your left knee and pull your left heel in toward your right buttock. Bend your right knee and place your right foot just beyond your left knee. Sit tall, pulling in your abs as you inhale and rotate to the right. Use your left hand, as shown, to gently pull your thigh. Hold 20 seconds, breathing deeply. Repeat on the other side, with your left leg on top.

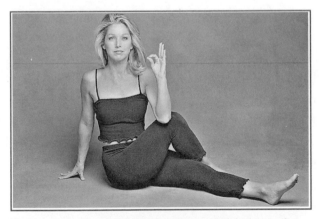

B. Next, extend your left leg and place your right foot to the outside of your left knee. Place your left elbow against your right thigh and twist to the right, as shown. Hold the pose for 20 seconds, breathing deeply. Repeat on the other side.

Benefits

This gently keeps your back muscles limber. A trunk rotation will help keep your back healthy, and it increases the suppleness of your vertebrae.

Pilates Pointers

► As you twist, extend through your crown, elongating your body as much as possible.

► Try to keep both buttocks firmly anchored to the floor.

► Use your right hand to press into the floor and keep your body upright, not leaning back.

My 5-MINUTE Balance Ball Routine

designed this routine for those who say, "I'd like to get in shape, but I just don't have the time." Well, if you don't have 10 minutes to spare, how about 5? You can do this while you're waiting for dinner to cook, while you're on hold on the phone (using a speakerphone), or even just as you roll out of bed.

This routine uses a large exercise ball, sometimes called a resistance ball or a stability ball. These large inflated balls force you to use your entire body and core abdominal muscles to stay balanced on the ball. It's an incredibly efficient, not to mention fun, form of exercise. And unlike a weight bench, the ball can double as a fun activity for your kids. My daughters love stretching and balancing on it.

Because you'll be using balance to stay propped on the ball, some of the following moves may feel awkward at first. Keep doing them. You'll soon get the hang of them!

Make each exercise last for about a minute. If you have to repeat the move on the other side of your body, then do 30 seconds for each side.

The Pushup

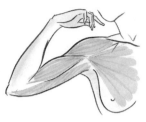

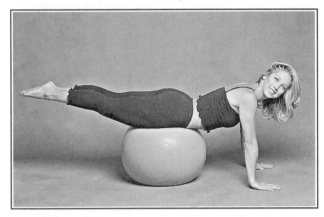

A. With your thighs, hips, and lower belly on the ball and your hands on the floor under your shoulders, extend your legs behind your body.

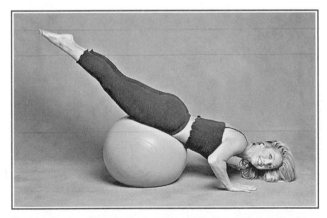

B. Keep your abs engaged and navel in toward your spine as you inhale, then bend your elbows and lower your chest to the floor, raising your legs up. Your body should form a straight line throughout the move. Exhale and press into your palms to raise yourself to the starting position. Repeat.

Benefits

This exercise targets your chest, arms, and shoulders while also targeting your abs, buttocks, and back for balance.

Pilates Pointers

► To keep your back from arching, press your belly button toward your spine and engage your abs.

► To firm up your chest more, just place your hands farther apart but still in line with your shoulders.

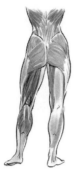

Benefit

This exercise targets the area of your lower buttocks that extends below your swimsuit.

Pilates Pointers

► Though your lower back will arch some during this move, attempt to keep it flat by pulling up and in with your abs. Remember your corset. Zip it up!

► Squeeze your buttocks.

Buttocks Firmer

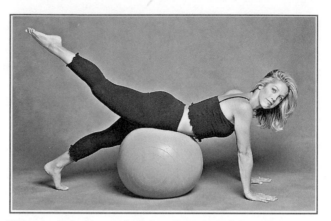

With your belly, hips, and thighs still on the ball from the previous move, your hands on the floor under your shoulders, and the balls of your feet on the floor, press your navel toward your spine as you inhale and extend your right leg up, as shown, feeling the movement in your lower right buttock. Lower as you exhale. Repeat for 30 seconds, then switch legs.

Denise-eology . . .

"Don't use time carelessly, for it can never be retrieved. Life is precious."

Outer Hip and Thigh Slimmer

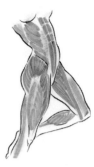

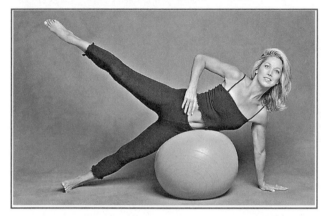

Adjust your body on the ball so that your outer left waist, hip, and ribs are on the ball. Place your left hand on the floor below your left shoulder. Extend your left leg and balance on the outer edge of your left foot. Place your right hand on your hip. Moving from your hips, inhale and raise your extended right leg up, as shown, then exhale as you lower. Repeat for 30 seconds, then switch sides.

Benefit
This targets the area of the outer thigh that's prone to "saddlebags."

Pilates Pointers
► Try to keep your hips stacked on top of each other rather than allowing your top hip to collapse forward.
► Open your chest.

Denise-eology . . .
"With Pilates, you feel invigorated, yet relaxed."

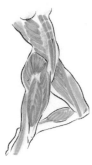

Inner Thigh Firmer

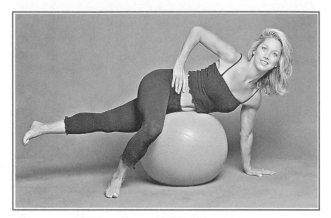

Benefit

This exercise firms up your inner thighs, preventing your thighs from rubbing together or jiggling when you walk.

Pilates Pointers

► To avoid the tendency to lean forward during the movement, place your top hand on your top hipbone.

► Keep your abs strong and your navel pulled in.

With your outer left torso on the ball in the same position as the previous exercise, bend your right leg and place your right foot on the floor close to the ball. Extend your left leg, inhale, and raise it, as shown, feeling the movement in your left inner thigh. Exhale as you lower. Repeat for 30 seconds, then switch sides.

Ab/Torso Toner

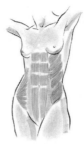

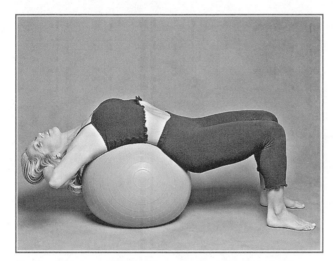

A. Lie with your middle and lower back and your buttocks on the ball with your knees bent and feet on the floor. Place your hands behind your head for support, with your elbows out to the sides. Press your navel in toward your spine as you lower your head and shoulders back, feeling a deep stretch from your pelvic bone to your neck.

Benefit

This strengthens and stretches your entire abdominal area.

Pilates Pointer

▶ Breathe deeply as you stretch back on the ball, exhaling with a sigh. Deep breaths will help to relax your back and allow you to surrender to gravity.

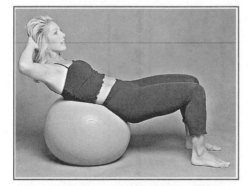

B. Keep your abs engaged as you exhale and curl your ribs toward your hipbones, scooping your belly into a C shape. Lower as you inhale. Repeat.

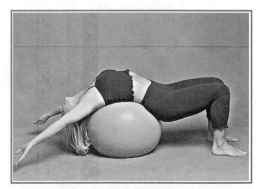

C. Finish by stretching out the front of your torso with your arms extended over your head and fingertips approaching the floor. Yes, this feels wonderful.

Part

4

YOUR 3-WEEK Total
Body MAKEOVER

A Progressive Plan for Complete
MIND-BODY
FITNESS

You'll be amazed at how much you can accomplish in just 21 days. You can stand up to an inch taller or lose an inch around your waist and thighs. You can feel more focused, energetic, coordinated, balanced, confident, smooth, flexible, and supple. Your aches and pains will start to diminish. Your stress will subside. In just 21 days, you'll create a new you. You'll have completely redefined your mind and body.

This 3-week plan works by combining the best of the Pilates method with a practical, nourishing eating plan; a fat-burning cardio routine; and my positive-thinking exercises. Together, these four elements work synergistically not only to help you make over your body but also to help you feel good for life. So to be most successful, you need to follow all four of the elements. I start you off slowly, and you progress gradually. Anyone can do it!

My Eating Plan. An indispensable part of your makeover, the tips, strategies, and sample menus in my eating plan will help you eat the right amount of calories to help you lose weight and keep it off. Suggesting small substitutions for breakfast, lunch, dinner, and snacks, the makeover plan will show you how to focus on the healthiest foods possible—ones that will increase your energy, helping you to look forward to your Pilates and cardio workouts. These foods also will help you look your best, giving your skin, face, and hair a healthy glow. And sticking with them will keep you healthy and vital from the inside out for decades to come.

Progressive Pilates. Three 15-minute sessions of Pilates a week will give you longer, leaner muscles; improve your posture; and relax your mind. The workouts in this section increase gradually in difficulty, starting at a level that anyone can tackle and advancing to an intermediate level. In each session, you will work your entire body, giving you a complete conditioning workout from your head to your toes.

My Cardio Program. Pilates does a wonderful job at strengthening and stretching all the muscles in your body. For optimal health and fat-burning, however, you must couple it with some type of cardio (aerobic) activity that increases your heart rate. My Cardio Program calls for three to four 20- to 30-minute sessions a week. You can choose from my walking program, my in-home cardio workout, or a variety of other options, in any combination. Whatever combination of activities you do will help you burn extra calories, control your appetite, and fight off age-related diseases such as heart disease.

My Positive-Thinking Program. I like to make every day my best day. I believe in being optimistic; it truly helps me to shed unnecessary stress. It also helps me avoid negative emotions that can gobble up so much time and energy. Positive thinking will do more than help you enjoy life to its fullest; it will also help you bring enthusiasm to everyone around you. A good attitude is contagious!

Everything You Need in One Step-by-Step Plan

When you combine Pilates with good nutrition, fat-burning cardio exercise, and positive-thinking habits, your body, your mind, and your life will undergo an amazing transformation, helping you to be the healthiest and happiest that you can be.

The 3-Week Total Body Makeover is perfect for anyone who needs a blueprint to lose weight. At times, we all need help to reach our goals. This plan provides step-by-step instructions. And the Personal 3-Week Makeover Diary at the end of this section enables you to track what you eat every day along with your Pilates sessions and cardio workouts. You will see results in just 3 weeks.

This program lasts 3 weeks because that's how long it takes to see noticeable changes in your body. Also, research shows that it takes 21 days to form a habit. So, while you may need a focused program to keep you motivated for the first 3 weeks of your new Pilates habit, you'll find yourself naturally gravitating to these workouts after you complete the program.

This makeover will take a commitment on your part. Can you commit to taking a close, honest look at your eating habits and making a few changes? Can you commit to three 15-minute sessions of Pilates a week as well as three to four 20- to 30-minute sessions of cardio exercise?

If you answer yes to both of these questions, then this is the right plan for you. Remember, embarking on this plan is worth it because you are worth it. You can do it!

Beyond 3 Weeks

Upon finishing the 3-Week Total Body Makeover, you'll be fit enough for any of the routines in this book, including the Complete Pilates Program in part 2. Choose the routines that you like the most. For example, you might mix it up, doing one of the routines in week 3 of this program one day and the Complete Pilates Program in part 2 for a subsequent session. Varying your workouts will keep you from getting bored with any one routine. I love changing my Pilates routines. It allows me to target different muscle groups during each workout, making each exercise session even more effective.

Which routine you choose is not as important as performing some form of Pilates at least three times a week. Continue with your cardio exercise three to four times a week and stick to your new eating habits. This is just the start of a complete body-maintenance program that you can use for the rest of your life. And it's the exact same maintenance plan that I personally use to stay fit and healthy!

Denise-eology . . .

"From your own efforts,
you will make a difference,
and you will feel good
about yourself."

My Eating PLAN

No health makeover would be complete without an eating plan, and my 3-Week Total Body Makeover is no exception. Following my sample menus, calorie guidelines, and food tips will provide more energy for your Pilates routines and help control your weight, but it will also protect against disease, keeping you healthy and vital for decades to come.

As a bonus, eating the right diet will give your skin a radiant glow.

Rest assured, making over your diet won't mean giving up all your favorite foods and living on nothing but celery and rice cakes. Nor will you have to load up on unfamiliar, hard-to-find health foods or spend hours in the kitchen (unless you want to). And you won't go hungry. People often tell me that they can't believe how much food I eat and still manage to stay trim. Here, you'll learn my eating secrets.

Where Do You Start?

Before you can figure out what to change, you need to review what you're eating now. Think about the meals and snacks you eat and serve your family in any given week. What does your menu look like?

Possibly as a result of our fast-paced lifestyles, so many of us get by on macaroni and cheese, frozen pizza, burgers, canned spaghetti and meatballs, and other foods that can be heated up quickly, making them incredibly convenient. Or we rely on snacks eaten right out of the box as pick-me-ups to get through the day. Yet convenience foods and snacks tend to be high in fat, starch, and calories, and they often lack the fiber, vitamins, minerals, and other nutrients you need to be your absolute best.

I developed my eating plan with Leslie Bonci, R.D., a nutritionist with whom I've worked for years. Without sacrificing convenience, my menu plans, tips, and strategies will help you make over your diet in three fundamental ways: substituting high-fiber foods for low-fiber foods, switching from harmful fats to healthful fats, and controlling your calories. It's that simple!

More Fiber, Please

Skins, seeds, husks, and other structural parts of fruits, vegetables, beans, peas, lentils, nuts, and seeds are carbohydrates that pass through your gastrointestinal tract undigested. Corn and grains like wheat, rice, oats, and barley are also high in fiber, provided their outer husks have not been removed in the course of being processed into bread, crackers, pasta, or cereals.

Fiber may pass through your system undigested, but it's far from useless. Fiber moves whatever you eat through your intestines, maintaining regular bowel function and keeping you regular. But fiber also prevents your body from absorbing some of the fat and calories from your food. In fact, each gram of fiber you eat can cancel out 9 calories from your calorie intake. My eating plan supplies 30 grams of fiber a day. That amounts to 270 calories that you eat but don't absorb.

Fiber also fills you up, allowing you to eat less food but still feel satisfied.

Switch to the Good Fats

Each gram of fat you eat, whether it's from an animal source (like meat, milk, eggs, or butter) or a plant source (like olive oil, peanuts, or avocados) contains 9 calories, period.

My eating plan emphasizes plant sources of fat over animal sources. Fats derived from animal sources are high in saturated fats, and evidence suggests they raise your risk of heart disease and cancer. (A few plant sources of fat, namely coconut oil and palm oil, are also high in saturated fat.) Similar evidence exists for what scientists call trans fatty acids—modified vegetable fats found in many margarines, shortening, crackers, chips, and other foods containing partially hydrogenated vegetable oil, which has been altered to remain solid at room temperature. So I don't eat any foods that list "partially hydrogenated oil" on the label. And naturally, I limit my intake of animal fats.

The exception is fish: Omega-3 fatty acids, found in deep-water fish like tuna and salmon, *lower* your risk for all types of disease, from heart disease to arthritis. Flaxseed oil also contains omega-3 fatty acids.

I also eat vegetable and nut oils in their natural form—canola oil, olive oil, nuts and nut oils, and other plant foods. Compared to animal fats, they're relatively low in saturated fat and high in monounsaturated fat, which is associated with heart health.

My eating plan is carefully designed to derive 25 percent of your calories from fat, focusing on the healthiest types.

Control Calories, Painlessly

No matter how you look at it, weight control comes down to one simple equation: calories consumed over calories burned. If you regularly eat more calories than you burn, you will gain weight. If you regularly burn more calories a day than you eat—through work, play, and exercise—you'll lose weight. If you equalize the calories you consume and the calories you burn every day, you'll maintain your weight. I've maintained my weight at around 118 pounds most of my adult life, except for when I was pregnant (when I gained 35 pounds with each baby).

I personally eat about 2,000 calories a day, but I'm active. My eating plan offers sample menus for three calorie levels, geared toward individual activity levels and weight goals.

The 1,350-Calorie Plan. This is perfect for women who want to lose weight, especially those who have desk jobs or do other sedentary work and who are getting the minimum amount of exercise (3 days a week) on the 3-Week Total Body Makeover plan. Don't be tempted to cut calories further, because your metabolism will automatically slow as your body attempts to conserve energy and calories.

Once you work up to the 20 to 30 minutes of cardio exercise three to four times a week, as suggested in My Cardio Program, you could move up to the 1,600-Calorie Plan. Some people who are just starting to work out or who carry a lot of extra weight might take a little longer than 3 weeks to work up to the full amount of exercise recommended.

The 1,600-Calorie Plan. This is designed for women and men who perform some type of cardio exercise—such as walking, jogging, or some other form of cardio 4 days a week as part of the makeover plan—and who also want to lose weight. This is also a great maintenance plan for keeping off weight.

The 2,200-Calorie Plan. This is for very active men and women who have active jobs—such as construction or waiting tables—or who are firmly committed to working out regularly, spending as much as an hour or more doing some form of cardio exercise 4 or more days of the week.

All three calorie plans are designed to help you lose about 2 pounds a week. Research has shown that rapid weight loss—more than 2 pounds a week—tends to come from muscle rather than fat. Losing weight more rapidly is tempting, but it slows your metabolism, quickly causing your weight-loss efforts to plateau. Losing weight gradually—2 pounds a week or less—takes patience, but it's the smart way to do it.

Slow weight loss tends to come exclusively from fat. And you'll be more likely to maintain your weight loss over a long period of time and not lose and regain the same 5, 10, or 20 pounds (or more) again and again.

At about 2 pounds a week, you can expect to lose 6 pounds on the 3-Week Total Body Makeover plan. To lose additional weight, continue following week 3 of the plan until you reach your goal, and then, of course, stick with it for life (and for good health).

Pick-Your-Calorie Plan

The following chart lists the number of servings to aim for on the 3-Week Total Body Makeover plan, depending on the calorie level that's appropriate for you.

Food Category	1,350 Calories	1,600 Calories	2,200 Calories
Fruits	2	3	4
Vegetables	3	4	5
Whole grains	6	6	9
Starch	1	2	3
Protein	2	2	2
Dairy	2	2	2
Fat	4	6	8
Water	8	8	8

Denise-eology . . .

"Sure, I like to pig out sometimes. But ultimately I feel much better when I eat healthy."

Tally Your Food

The three calorie plans above and the convenient yet wholesome menus that follow focus on foods from seven categories—fruits, vegetables, whole grains, starch, protein, dairy, and fat—plus water. I've found that putting food into those categories helps me to visualize my nutritional goals for the day. Rather than counting every single calorie I put in my mouth, I merely have to keep a mental tab of how many servings of fruit or dairy or protein I've had in a day. (I eat somewhere between 1,600 and 2,200 calories.) This mental tab helps keep me from going overboard on unhealthy foods as well as helps me remember to pile on the healthy ones. You can keep track of your daily totals in the Personal 3-Week Makeover Diary at the end of this section.

On my eating plan, fruits, vegetables, and whole grains will make up more than half of your new diet, and for good reason.

Fruits and Vegetables

Naturally low in calories, fruits and vegetables allow you to eat more food while still losing weight. Consuming five or more servings of fruits or vegetables a day is part of my secret for staying trim. I always "strive for five."

Fruits and vegetables are nutrition powerhouses. Research has found that the deep pigments that give dark-colored fruits and vegetables their color—for example, the lycopene that makes tomatoes red—supply benefits beyond what vitamins and minerals provide. Research studies show that substances called phytochemicals in these plant pigments help to prevent heart disease and cancer.

Start with breakfast—and keep going. For me, morning is the easiest time to get in one or two servings of fruits or vegetables. For example, I sometimes mix berries or sliced fruit into my cereal or into fat-free plain yogurt. If I'm making an omelet, I make sure to add at least three different types of vegetables to the eggs so that it's chock full of onions, tomatoes, and mushrooms, for example.

At midmorning, I usually follow up with a fruit snack of a banana, apple, orange, half a grapefruit, or berries.

At lunch, I squeeze in more veggies by eating a spinach salad; making a spinach, tomato, and turkey sandwich; or having vegetable soup. (Because soup takes time to eat, it helps slow you down, preventing you from overeating.) At dinner, I try to get two more vegetables, such as steamed broccoli and asparagus.

Create a rainbow on your plate. When choosing vegetables for soups, salads, or side dishes, think "color." Different-colored fruits and vegetables give you a great variety of nutrients and create a prettier plate of food.

Whole Grains and Starches

Whole grain breads and pastas, along with unprocessed grains like brown rice, oatmeal, quinoa, and barley provide fiber to fill you up as well as an array of nutrients to keep you healthy and energized. In contrast, processed starch such as white pasta, white rice, and crackers provide very little in the way of fiber or nutrients. Yet they're difficult to avoid completely. I try to eat as few processed starches as possible, selecting whole grains instead. My plan shows you how to do that.

To maximize your intake of whole grains and minimize the amount of processed grains and starch you eat, try the following suggestions.

Read labels closely when shopping. Look for foods that contain at least 3 grams of fiber per serving. For example, my favorite breakfast cereal, Kashi, is made from fiber-rich whole grains. It also contains no preservatives and offers a touch of satisfying protein. I eat it many mornings for breakfast along with fat-free milk and sliced fruit.

Try 50/50. Like many children, my daughters, Katie and Kelly, don't like the taste or texture of many types of whole grains. So I meet them halfway. For example, to get them to eat brown rice, I started by serving brown and white rice mixed together. Once my kids got used to that mixture, I began adding more and more brown rice and decreasing the amount of white rice. Now my girls eat 100 percent brown rice.

Add extra flavor. Boil rice in fat-free chicken broth with a little water.

Proteins

An essential nutrient for life, protein is a primary component of the brain, heart, blood, skin, and hair. Your body also needs and uses protein to build and repair muscle, an important benefit when you exercise regularly. Protein can also help fill you up, which will keep you from overeating.

If you're like many people, you get most of your protein from animal sources such as meat, poultry, and dairy. Unfortunately, animal sources of protein also tend to contain artery-clogging saturated fat. Instead, try to select plant sources of protein like beans, peas, and lentils, which contain a lot of fiber with no fat. (Grains, too, supply some protein, but not nearly as much as beans.)

Here are some tips to help you make smart protein choices.

Sneak beans into your meals. I always toss chickpeas and kidney beans in my soups, salads, and meat chili, for example.

Substitute soy foods for meat when possible. Soybeans truly are a wonder food. Research shows that eating soy regularly can lower cholesterol levels, reduce cancer risk, build stronger bones, and possibly even reduce menopausal symptoms such as hot flashes in women.

And soy is naturally low in calories, making it a perfect choice for your makeover plan. Consider using soy sausage, patties, hot dogs, and ground veggie round in place of beef or pork versions. Also miso, a grainy paste made from soybeans, is an excellent ingredient for marinades and sauces. (I'm trying to get used to it, too!)

For a quick, nutritious pick-me-up, try soy nuts. These roasted soybeans taste great.

Eat fish twice a week. Most types of fish are naturally low in fat and calories. Deep-water fish such as tuna, salmon, and mackerel are stellar choices, given the omega-3 fats they supply. So I try to have fish twice a week: once for dinner and then a tuna sandwich for lunch on a different day. For dinner, I'll broil salmon for my husband and me and simultaneously bake breaded fish for the kids. (I'm still trying to get my girls to appreciate fish. Baked breaded fish is definitely a step up from fish sticks.) To cut down on the fat in my tuna sandwich, I buy water-packed tuna and mix some mustard, vinegar, relish, or other fat-free condiments in with the mayonnaise. That way, I need only a tad of mayo but still end up with a great-tasting sandwich.

Choose the leanest cuts of meat. Beef eye round, top round, flank steak, pork tenderloin, lamb foreshank, and veal leg make excellent choices. They have no more than 25 to 30 percent of calories from fat. Ground top round (97 percent lean) and ground sirloin (90 percent lean) are better choices than ground round (85 percent lean) and regular ground beef (73 percent lean). For other cuts, trim off any visible fat.

Use skinless chicken and turkey. I often use ground turkey breast instead of ground beef to make spaghetti sauce, tacos, sloppy joes, and chili.

Dairy Products

Milk and other dairy products are rich sources of calcium, an important bone-building mineral. Without enough calcium, men and women alike run the risk of developing weak, brittle bones that fracture easily with age.

All animal products, however, including dairy, contain some artery-clogging saturated fat. Eliminate as much of this fat as possible by choosing the lowest-fat dairy products you can find.

Opt for fat-free milk, low-fat yogurt, and low-fat cottage cheese. They supply you with bone-building calcium, and they double as a great protein source. They're also convenient. When I'm on the run, I take a container of low-fat cottage cheese or yogurt with me and eat it on the go.

Snack on string cheese. A type of mozzarella, low-fat string cheese makes a great snack, particularly for kids. When my girls come home from school and want a snack, we often have a little string cheese together.

Fats

Fat helps you to feel full, makes food taste good, and helps you to absorb fat-soluble vitamins A, D, E, and K. Here's what I do to eat more of the healthy fats and less of the others.

Read the ingredient list for every type of food that comes in a box or bag. Look for the words "partially hydrogenated oil"—a code phrase for trans fatty acids, which you want to avoid. You can find crackers, breakfast cereals, and other convenience foods (including some margarines) that do not contain this kind of fat.

Favor avocados, olives, peanut butter, and nuts. The monounsaturated fats they supply will help protect you against heart disease.

Use olive oil and canola oil in cooking, in salads, and on bread. Keep butter and margarine (a common source of trans fatty acids) to a minimum.

Try flaxseed oil on your salads. You'll get a healthy dose of heart-healthy omega-3 fatty acids. (You can buy flaxseed oil at health food stores.)

Snack on nuts. I like to make my own trail mix, combining raw almonds with dried fruit and whole grain breakfast cereal and tossing it into little plastic bags that I stash in my purse to eat when I'm on the go. This little emergency snack will help keep you from relying on vending machines or reaching for chips as your afternoon snack.

Water

Although water contains no calories, it helps contribute to a feeling of fullness, especially when you drink some right before meals. And your body needs water for countless processes, from food digestion to temperature regulation. Also, because your brain and blood are largely made of water, a shortfall of fluid can make you feel tired, sluggish, and dull—which is no way to begin a Pilates session. So my plan calls for eight 8-ounce glasses of water a day.

I personally drink five small bottled waters or two 1-liter bottles every day. I carry them with me and aim to return home with them empty. I stash bottled water everywhere—in my purse, in my car, in my office, and in various rooms in the house. That way, I always have a bottle to sip from, no matter how harried my day. Being prepared is the best way to truly ensure that you drink the 64 ounces of water recommended each day.

One way to tell if you're drinking enough water is by checking your urine color. If it's very pale yellow, you're doing great. If it's bright yellow or deep gold, you need more fluid.

To ensure that you get enough water, try the following tips.

Drink two glasses as soon as you get up in the morning. After sleeping for 7 to 8 hours, your body is dehydrated, and you need water in the morning.

Drink a glass of water before each meal and one with meals. That will help you to automatically eat less.

Substitute water for other drinks. Soft drinks and juice drinks contain calories from sugar. Water is a better choice—and it's calorie-free.

How Much Is a Serving?

I travel a lot, and my husband I and like to dine out with friends. So I eat my share of meals away from home. I notice that restaurant portions tend to be huge. And snack foods and beverages all seem to come in jumbo size. So it's easy to lose sight of what a normal portion of food looks like.

Here's a quick guide to what constitutes a basic serving on my eating plan, to keep you from unwittingly exceeding your daily calorie limit. Amounts on the 7-Day Menu Plan may sometimes vary according to the calorie level followed. Pay special attention to serving sizes for starches and fats.

Fruits: 1 medium-size piece of fruit (apple, orange), ½ grapefruit, 1 slice or 1 cup cubed melon (cantaloupe, honeydew), 1¼ cups cubed watermelon, ¾ cup berries, 12 cherries, 15 grapes, 2 figs, 1 kiwifruit, ⅛ avocado, ½ cup chopped mango, 2 prunes, ⅓ cup raisins or dried fruit, 1 small or ½ large banana, ½ cup canned or frozen fruit, ½ cup fruit juice

Fruit juice also counts as ½ serving of water. Avocado doubles as one serving of fat.

Vegetables: ½ cup vegetables (fresh or frozen, cooked or raw), 1 large lettuce leaf or other salad greens, 1 slice tomato, 3 or 4 carrot sticks, 1 cup cooked squash, ¾ cup vegetable juice or vegetable soup

Whole grains: ⅓ cup cooked brown rice; ½ cup cooked whole grain such as barley or bulgur; ½ cup granola; ½ whole grain bagel, roll, or English muffin; 1 slice 100 percent whole grain bread; 1 whole wheat pita; ½ cup hot whole grain cereal; ¾ cup cold whole grain cereal; 3 tablespoons wheat germ; 2½ tablespoons whole wheat flour; ½ cup whole wheat pasta or spelt or millet noodles

Starch: ⅓ cup white rice, ½ cup cooked white pasta, 1 small potato, ½ cup mashed potatoes, 1 medium ear corn on the cob, ½ cup cooked corn, 3 tablespoons cornmeal, 4 cups popcorn, 3 graham crackers, 3 ounces corn chips or potato chips

Unless they are made fat-free, fatty starches such as biscuits, corn bread, muffins, taco shells, and chips also double as one serving of fat.

Protein: 2 ounces fish or seafood, 2 ounces lean meat or chicken or turkey with no skin, 2 ounces luncheon meat, 1 egg, 4 egg whites, ½ cup cooked beans or lentils, ½ cup cooked soybeans, 1 soy burger, 1 ounce soy cheese, 1 soy hot dog, 8 ounces soy milk, ½ cup tofu (soft or firm)

Fatty cuts of meat (beef, pork), fatty types of fish (salmon, sardines), and full-fat luncheon meats also count as one serving of fat.

Dairy: 1 cup fat-free milk, low-fat buttermilk, or fat-free yogurt; ½ cup cottage cheese; 2 ounces cheese

Dairy also counts as one serving of protein. Full-fat cheese also counts as one serving of fat. Milk and soy milk also count as one serving of water.

Fat: 1 teaspoon olive, canola, flaxseed, or other vegetable oil; 8 large olives; 1 teaspoon walnut or other nut oil; 2 tablespoons nuts; 2 teaspoons peanut butter or other nut butter; 1 tablespoon pumpkin or sunflower seeds; 1 teaspoon butter; 1 teaspoon margarine; 1 teaspoon full-fat mayonnaise; 1 tablespoon full-fat cream cheese or sour cream; 2 tablespoons half-and-half

Water: 8 ounces water or herbal tea

Denise's 7-Day Menu Plan

To show exactly how my food tallies and serving tips translate into real meals, nutritionist Leslie Bonci, R.D., and I designed seven sample menus. Try to follow this menu for week 1. If you truly don't like something or if you go out for lunch or dinner, you may substitute similar foods. To keep to the calorie count, stick to the portions stated. And make sure you eat your veggies!

This should help you get an idea of how to balance your day-to-day menus for weeks 2 and 3 of the plan and beyond. (And of course, if you're cooking for yourself and others, multiple the quantities shown by the number of people served.)

Day 1

Menu	1,350	1,600	2,200
		Calorie Levels	
BREAKFAST			
Fat-free milk	1 cup	1 cup	1 cup
Flake cereal (Kashi)	2¼ cups	2¼ cups	2¼ cups
Whole wheat toast	—	1 slice	1 slice
Butter or trans-free margarine	—	2 tsp	2 tsp
Orange juice	½ cup	½ cup	½ cup
LUNCH			
Ham and Cheese Sandwich:			
Sliced lean ham	2 oz	2 oz	2 oz
Low-fat cheese	2 slices	2 slices	2 slices
Spinach	1 large leaf	1 large leaf	1 large leaf
Tomato	1 slice	1 slice	1 slice
Mayonnaise	2 tsp	2 tsp	2 tsp
Rye bread	2 slices	2 slices	2 slices
Carrot sticks	—	4	4
Baked tortilla chips	—	—	1½ oz
Fresh peach	1	1	1
SNACK			
Chocolate pudding (made with fat-free milk)	½ cup	½ cup	½ cup
Ripe banana	—	1 small	1 small
DINNER			
Stir-Fry:*			
Cubed turkey breast	2 oz	2 oz	2 oz
Chopped garlic	1 tsp	1 tsp	1 tsp
Chopped fresh ginger	½ tsp	½ tsp	½ tsp
Mixed veggies (cabbage, mushrooms, snow peas, red pepper)	1 cup	1 cup	1½ cups
Sesame oil	2 tsp	2 tsp	4 tsp
Mandarin oranges	—	—	½ cup
Soy sauce	To taste	To taste	To taste
Cooked brown rice	⅔ cup	⅔ cup	1 cup

*In a lightly oiled nonstick skillet, sauté the turkey breast over medium heat for 6 to 8 minutes, or until cooked through. Stir in the garlic and ginger. Add the vegetables. Cook, stirring constantly until the veggies are crisp-tender. Toss with the sesame oil and oranges. Add the soy sauce to taste. Serve over rice.

Day 2

Menu	1,350	1,600	2,200
		Calorie Levels	

BREAKFAST

Breakfast Sandwich:

	1,350	1,600	2,200
Low-fat cheese	1½ oz	1½ oz	1½ oz
Whole grain English muffin	1	2	2
Fresh pear	1	1	1

LUNCH

Roast Beef Sandwich:

	1,350	1,600	2,200
Sliced lean roast beef	2 oz	2 oz	2 oz
Spinach	1 large leaf	1 large leaf	1 large leaf
Tomato	1 slice	1 slice	1 slice
Mayonnaise	1 tsp	1 tsp	1 tsp
Multigrain bread	2 slices	2 slices	2 slices
Pretzels	—	—	1½ oz
Fat-free plain yogurt	1 cup	1 cup	1 cup
Kiwifruit	1	1	1

SNACK

	1,350	1,600	2,200
Gingersnaps	3	3	3
Pineapple juice	—	½ cup	½ cup

DINNER

Grilled Tuna Steaks:*

	1,350	1,600	2,200
Tuna steak	2 oz	2 oz	2 oz
Sweet Rainbow Salsa**	½ cup	½ cup	½ cup
Whole grain sandwich roll	1	1	1

Salad:

	1,350	1,600	2,200
Mesclun greens	2 cups	2 cups	2 cups
Olive oil	1 tsp	1 tsp	2 tsp
Grated carrots and sliced mushrooms	—	—	1 cup
Pine nuts	—	—	1 Tbsp
Baked beans	—	—	⅓ cup
Fresh mango	—	—	½ cup

*Brush the tuna with 1 Tbsp prepared barbecue sauce. Grill until the steaks flake easily when tested with a fork, about 2 minutes per side. Place steak on a sandwich roll and spoon some salsa on top of the tuna.

**For salsa, cook 1 chopped onion in a nonstick skillet over medium heat. Stir until the onion is tender, adding water if needed to prevent sticking. Add 3 Tbsp balsamic vinegar, 2 medium chopped tomatoes, 1 chopped sweet green pepper, 1 chopped sweet yellow pepper. Cook for 5 minutes. Stir in 2 Tbsp chopped fresh cilantro, 1 Tbsp chopped fresh basil, and 1 small overripe chopped banana.

Day 3

Menu	1,350	1,600	2,200
		Calorie Levels	
BREAKFAST			
Fat-free plain yogurt	8 oz	8 oz	8 oz
Low-fat granola	¾ cup	1 cup	1¼ cups
Fresh blueberries	¾ cup	¾ cup	¾ cup
Chopped walnuts	—	8 halves	8 halves
LUNCH			
Turkey Sandwich:			
Sliced turkey breast	2 oz	2 oz	2 oz
Low-fat cheese	1½ oz	1½ oz	1½ oz
Alfalfa sprouts	½ cup	½ cup	½ cup
Romaine lettuce	1 large leaf	1 large leaf	1 large leaf
Tomato	1 slice	1 slice	1 slice
Olive oil	2 tsp	2 tsp	2 tsp
Whole wheat pita	1	1	2
Plums	2 small	2 small	2 small
SNACK			
Fat-free potato chips	1½ oz	1½ oz	1½ oz
Grapefruit juice	—	½ cup	1 cup
DINNER			
Tortilla Scramble:*			
Chopped fresh veggies of your choice	1 cup	1 cup	1 cup
Chopped garlic, diced onions, diced hot pepper, and ground cumin	To taste	To taste	To taste
Egg whites	4	4	4
6-inch whole grain tortilla	1	1	2
Black beans, canned	½ cup	½ cup	½ cup
Reduced-fat sour cream	3 Tbsp	3 Tbsp	3 Tbsp
Pineapple chunks	—	—	½ cup
Tossed salad greens	1 large leaf	1 large leaf	1 large leaf
Olive oil	1 tsp	1 tsp	1 tsp

*In a nonstick skillet over medium heat, stir-fry the vegetables along with the garlic, onions, hot pepper, and cumin for 5 to 6 minutes, or until the vegetables are tender. In a bowl, combine the egg whites with ¼ cup water, then whisk until the whites foam. Pour over the vegetables. Cover and reduce heat to low. Allow it to stand, without stirring, until cooked through, about 5 minutes. Spoon into the tortilla with black beans and sour cream.

Day 4

Menu	1,350	1,600	2,200
		Calorie Levels	

BREAKFAST

	1,350	1,600	2,200
Graham crackers	3	6	6
Peanut butter	—	2 tsp	2 tsp
Flake cereal (like Kashi)	¾ cup	¾ cup	1½ cups
Fat-free milk	½ cup	½ cup	1 cup
Grapefruit or orange	½	½	½

LUNCH

	1,350	1,600	2,200
Grilled Chicken Salad:			
Tossed salad greens	1 large leaf	1 large leaf	1 large leaf
Olive oil	1 tsp	1 tsp	1 tsp
Grilled chicken	2 oz	2 oz	2 oz
Low-fat Jarlsberg cheese	1½ oz	1½ oz	1½ oz
Avocado	⅛	⅛	⅛
Whole wheat crackers	1½ oz	1½ oz	3 oz
Nectarine	1	1	1

SNACK

	1,350	1,600	2,200
Fat-free ice cream	½ cup	½ cup	½ cup
Cubed cantaloupe	—	1 cup	1 cup

DINNER

	1,350	1,600	2,200
Pasta Toss:*			
Olive oil	2 tsp	2 tsp	4 tsp
Chopped garlic	1 clove	1 clove	1 clove
Tomato sauce	½ cup	½ cup	¾ cup
Anise seed	⅛ tsp	⅛ tsp	⅛ tsp
Shredded fresh basil	2 leaves	2 leaves	2 leaves
Cayenne	Dash	Dash	Dash
Cannellini beans	½ cup	½ cup	½ cup
Cooked whole wheat pasta	½ cup	½ cup	¾ cup
Steamed broccoli with lemon juice	½ cup	½ cup	½ cup
Shredded leafy spinach	2 cups	2 cups	2 cups
Fat-free Italian dressing	1 Tbsp	1 Tbsp	1 Tbsp
Fresh apricots	—	—	2

*Sauté the garlic and olive oil in a heavy nonstick pan on medium-low heat for 1 minute or less, or until the garlic is soft but not brown. Stir in the tomato sauce. Add the anise seed, basil, and cayenne pepper. Simmer 2 to 3 minutes. Stir in the beans. Cover and simmer for 2 to 3 minutes, or until the beans are heated through. Serve over pasta.

Day 5

Menu	1,350	1,600	2,200
		Calorie Levels	
BREAKFAST			
Whole grain bagel	½	½	1
Low-fat Muenster cheese	1½ oz	1½ oz	1½ oz
Orange juice	½ cup	½ cup	½ cup
LUNCH			
Egg Salad Sandwich:			
Chopped hard-boiled egg	1	1	1
Mayonnaise	2 tsp	2 tsp	2 tsp
Minced celery	¼ cup	¼ cup	¼ cup
Sliced radishes	¼ cup	¼ cup	¼ cup
Chopped cucumber	¼ cup	¼ cup	¼ cup
Whole wheat pita	1	1	1
Romaine lettuce	1 large leaf	1 large leaf	1 large leaf
Fat-free vanilla yogurt	½ cup	½ cup	½ cup
Fresh raspberries	¾ cup	¾ cup	¾ cup
SNACK			
Low-fat popcorn	4 cups	4 cups	4 cups
Grape juice	—	½ cup	½ cup
DINNER			
Poached Salmon:*			
Salmon fillet	2 oz	2 oz	2 oz
Red-skinned potato, microwaved or baked	1 small	1 small	2 small
Green Beans:**			
Cut green beans	1 cup	1 cup	1½ cups
Chopped onion	¼ cup	¼ cup	¼ cup
Butter or trans-free margarine	1 tsp	2 tsp	4 tsp
Whole grain dinner roll	1	1	1
Fresh blueberries	—	—	¾ cup

*Cook the salmon skin side down in a heavy nonstick skillet over medium heat. Pour enough red wine over the salmon to almost cover it. Cook for 6 to 8 minutes, or until the salmon flakes easily when tested with a fork and the wine is almost gone. Season with salt and pepper.

**Sauté the green beans with the onion and margarine for 4 to 5 minutes, or until tender.

Day 6

Menu	1,350	1,600	2,200
	Calorie Levels		

BREAKFAST

	1,350	1,600	2,200
Oatmeal, cooked	1 cup	1 cup	1½ cups
Raisins	2 Tbsp	2 Tbsp	2 Tbsp
Chopped pecans	—	½ oz	½ oz
Whole wheat toast	1 slice	2 slices	2 slices
Fat-free milk	½ cup	½ cup	¾ cup

LUNCH

	1,350	1,600	2,200
Low-fat soy hot dog	1	1	1
Fat-free cheese	2 oz	2 oz	2 oz
Whole grain roll	1	1	1
Shredded cabbage and carrots	½ cup	½ cup	1 cup
Fat-free coleslaw dressing	1 Tbsp	1 Tbsp	1 Tbsp
Cubed watermelon	1¼ cups	1¼ cups	1¼ cups
Fat-free potato chips	—	—	1½ oz

SNACK

	1,350	1,600	2,200
Teddy Graham crackers	18	18	18
Blended fruit juice	—	½ cup	½ cup

DINNER

	1,350	1,600	2,200
Dijon Chicken:*			
Chicken breast	2 oz	2 oz	2 oz
Mashed potatoes	½ cup	½ cup	1 cup
Reduced-fat sour cream	3 Tbsp	3 Tbsp	3 Tbsp
Whole grain dinner roll	1	1	1
Butter or trans-free margarine	1 tsp	1 tsp	1 tsp
Spinach:**			
Steamed leaf spinach	½ cup	½ cup	½ cup
Yellow raisins	—	—	⅓ cup
Olive oil	—	—	2 tsp
Red-leaf lettuce	2 cups	2 cups	2 cups
Fat-free Catalina dressing	1 Tbsp	1 Tbsp	1 Tbsp
Artichoke hearts, canned in water	—	—	2

*Brush both sides of a boneless, skinless chicken breast with Dijon mustard. Place on a broiler pan covered with aluminum foil that has been lightly coated with cooking spray. Broil 4 minutes per side, or until the chicken is cooked through and the juices run clear.

**Toss the yellow raisins and olive oil with spinach, if allowed.

Day 7

Menu	1,350	1,600	2,200
		Calorie Levels	
BREAKFAST			
Low-fat waffles	2	4	5
Fat-free vanilla yogurt	½ cup	½ cup	½ cup
Applesauce with dash of cinnamon	½ cup	½ cup	½ cup
LUNCH			
Tuna Sandwich:			
Canned tuna, water-packed	2 oz	2 oz	2 oz
Mayonnaise	2 tsp	2 tsp	2 tsp
Celery, chopped	1 Tbsp	1 Tbsp	1 Tbsp
Lettuce	1 large leaf	1 large leaf	1 large leaf
Pumpernickel bread	2 slices	2 slices	2 slices
Vegetable soup	½ cup	1 cup	1 cup
Pretzels	—	—	1½ oz
Fat-free plain yogurt	½ cup	½ cup	½ cup
Fresh cherries	12	12	12
SNACK			
Reduced-fat frozen yogurt	¾ cup	¾ cup	¾ cup
Fresh strawberries	—	1¼ cups	1¼ cups
DINNER			
Grilled Pork Loin:*			
Pork tenderloin, center cut	2 oz	2 oz	2 oz
Mixed vegetables, cooked	½ cup	½ cup	½ cup
Corn on the cob	1 medium	1 medium	1 medium
Whole grain dinner roll	1	1	2
Butter or trans-free margarine	½ tsp	½ tsp	2½ tsp
Cubed watermelon	—	—	1¼ cups

*Brush the pork tenderloin with 1 Tbsp barbecue sauce. Grill, turning every 5 minutes until done (about 20 minutes total).

An Eating Plan for Life

The Food Tips of the Week in the 3-Week Makeover plan will help you adopt this eating plan quickly and make it a part of your life. And using the Personal 3-Week Makeover Diary at the end of this section will enable you to keep track of everything you eat (along with your Pilates sessions, walking workouts, and cardio exercises). Here are some additional tips for adopting the plan and sticking with it.

Eat often. People often comment about how often I eat. They can't figure out how I stay so fit when they always see me munching. Yet, surprisingly, munching is one of my secrets to staying trim. It's what you choose to eat that's important.

When you eat, your metabolism revs up, burning calories simply to digest your food. Snacking capitalizes on this metabolism boost by keeping that digestion-induced calorie burn running almost constantly. Also, snacking keeps you from becoming ravenous. A midmorning and midafternoon snack can take the edge off your appetite, preventing cravings and helping you to avoid overeating especially at dinner.

For my midmorning snack, I like to have some type of fruit around 10:30 A.M. I eat my afternoon snack with my girls when they come home from school at 3:00 P.M. I choose fun, low-fat foods that provide satisfying protein, such as string cheese (mentioned earlier), low-fat mozzarella sticks, or whole grain crackers with peanut butter.

Follow my 80 percent rule. My kids love desserts and treats, and though I want them to eat as healthfully as possible, I'm certainly not rigid about what they eat. In fact, I sometimes indulge with them.

To keep sweets and other treats from getting out of control, however, I enforce what I call the 80/20 rule. Eighty percent of the food we eat must be wholesome and nutritious, whereas 20 percent can come from favorite treats like dessert or snack foods. My kids are more likely to try new vegetables that I serve on their dinner plates if they know those veggies are their ticket to some ice cream later.

Introduce new foods. If my girls had their way, our family

Make Every Calorie Count

To help you visualize ways to make over your diet, take a look at the food substitutions shown here, which transform meals heavy in starch and fat into meals centered on fruits, vegetables, and high-fiber, low-fat whole grains. Then think about your own meal choices and make every calorie count. For every meal and snack, think about what you are eating. Are you making the healthiest food choice that you can? Could you sneak in more veggies or fruits? Does your plate resemble a rainbow with different-colored fruits and vegetables? Are you eating the leanest types of meat and dairy?

Before	After
BREAKFAST	
1 white bagel, large	½ whole grain bagel
Full-fat cream cheese	Low-fat cream cheese
	Fresh fruit
Regular latte	Latte made with fat-free milk
LUNCH	
Sub sandwich with Italian cold cuts on white roll	½ turkey and spinach sandwich on whole wheat bread or pita
	1 cup vegetable soup
DINNER	
Full plate (2 cups) white pasta with meat sauce	½ plate (½ cup) whole wheat pasta with ground turkey sauce
	1 green salad
	1 vegetable
SNACKS	
Potato chips	Apple
Premium ice cream	Fat-free frozen yogurt

would eat either pizza or macaroni and cheese for dinner every single night. Not only does eating the same foods all the time deprive your body of the array of nutrients that you need, it's also boring.

My girls don't always like every new food I serve. That's okay, but I want them to try it before declaring it "yucky." So we play a little game. I tell the girls that they have to eat as many bites of the new food as their age. That means Katie must take 8 bites and Kelly take 11 bites. Even though they try to take the smallest bites possible, this game encourages them to try new foods. My girls were surprised to learn that, after taking their 8 to 11 bites, broccoli wasn't so bad after all!

Put a curfew on your kitchen. Mindless late-night munching in front of the TV can add up to a lot of excess calories. Also, if you've had your midafternoon snack and a satisfying, fiber-rich dinner, you really shouldn't feel hungry in the evening, which means you're probably eating only out of boredom or habit. So I personally put an 8:00 P.M. curfew on my kitchen. I shut the kitchen doors and turn off the lights. I try to brush my teeth right away. The minty flavor of toothpaste keeps me from remotely feeling tempted to snack. Then, we take our dog, Madonna, for a walk.

Denise-eology . . .

"Eating right isn't about willpower; it's about changing bad habits."

My
Cardio
PROGRAM

Practicing Pilates three times a week takes care of two essential components of fitness: muscle toning and stretching. To become truly fit and healthy, however, you must combine Pilates with some type of cardiovascular—or "cardio"—exercise that gets your heart pumping, such as walking, running, biking, swimming, or rowing.

Also called aerobic exercise, your cardio routine will help you burn off excess fat. To lose 2 pounds a week, you need to consume 500 fewer calories than you burn a day. For example, exercising to my 45-minute *Ultimate Fat Burner* video can burn 500 calories in one session. After one cardio workout like that, you've already met your 500-calorie-a-day target reduction!

Cardio exercise helps shed fat in numerous other ways. Your metabolism stays charged for up to 3 hours after a cardio workout, so you continue to burn more calories after you've finished exercising. Also, research shows that regular doses of cardio exercise help to regulate your appetite. Finally, when you exercise regularly, your body redistributes stored fat, moving some fat into your muscles for easy access. That allows you to burn more fat during each exercise session.

Even if burning fat isn't a major concern for you, you need cardio to condition your heart and lungs and keep you healthy. A fit and well-conditioned heart is the center of a healthy body. Remember, your heart is muscle, too, so keep it pumping! Cardio also improves blood flow through your arteries and even encourages your body to build new capillaries. Because your blood carries energizing oxygen and nutrients to every cell in your body, cardio also gives you more stamina for everyday life.

My 3-Week Total Body Makeover calls for 3 to 4 days of cardio exercise a week. Numerous studies show that 3 days of cardio will condition your body, prevent heart disease, and lower blood pressure and cholesterol levels—and that's the amount of exercise the American College of Sports Medicine recommends, too.

If you want to lose weight, however, be sure to get in 4 days of cardio per week, rather than 3. Research has found that it takes a minimum of 2 hours of cardio exercise a week to lose weight and keep it off. The 3-week plan achieves that, working up to four sessions of 30 minutes each in week 3.

Choose a type of exercise that fits your schedule. For example, most mornings I wake up and go for a 20- to 30-minute walk. When I return, I do Pilates. I like the way walking warms my body, increasing blood circulation to my muscles, helping them to stretch more easily during my Pilates session.

If you don't have time to do cardio and Pilates back to back, try them on alternate days, doing Pilates on Mondays, Wednesdays, and Fridays and cardio on Tuesdays, Thursdays, and Saturdays, for example. Or you can walk in the morning and do Pilates at night. In other words, do what works for you. Keep track of your walking and cardio workouts and your Pilates sessions in the Personal 3-Week Makeover Diary at the end of this section.

Another great idea: Find a friend to be your cardio partner. Every

Sunday, I call my girlfriends to find out their schedules for the week. I try to make walking dates with as many as possible. That way I *know* I'll do it. I'm much less likely to skip my walk/run when I know I'll be disappointing someone else. It's a great way to catch up with my girlfriends during the walk. As we chat, the walk just flies by, and before we know it, we've walked for half an hour or even an hour.

Don't Forget to Warm Up and Cool Down

During each cardio session, remember to warm up and cool down for at least 5 minutes each. Your warmup does just that. It slowly increases your heart rate, getting more blood to your muscles to ready them for your workout. Your cooldown allows your heart to slow down gradually.

Your warmup and cooldown don't have to be complicated. They merely involve going a little slower than usual. For example, if you're walking, start at a leisurely pace for 5 to 6 minutes, and then pick up the pace by pumping your arms.

Here, I offer two specific cardio workouts, a walking program and an in-home cardio routine. Or you can try one of the cardio activities in "Other Great Cardio Workouts" on page 244. When you select an activity, choose one that you enjoy and that best suits your lifestyle and schedule.

Denise-eology . . .

"If you want to burn fat, you must do cardio. You're burning fat; you're burning butter."

My Walking Program

Walking is the best cardio choice for beginners because you need minimal equipment and expertise. It's one of the easiest forms of exercise to tailor to your schedule. And because walking places weight on your joints, it strengthens your bones, helping to protect against fractures associated with osteoporosis later in life.

Most people can walk without discomfort, which is a big plus. One exception: It's not always the best choice for those with arthritis. If that's the case for you, swimming or water aerobics might be a better option.

Turn Idle Time into Toning Time

Though I aim for 30 minutes of official exercise a day, I never miss an opportunity to move. I call these little 1-minute exercise bursts "fidgetcize," and I truly rely on them to help keep me trim and toned, particularly when I know I'll be spending much of the day on the phone.

Research has shown that little bursts of activity throughout the day can increase your calorie burn up to a startling 500 calories or more *per day*. And these little bursts are simple and easy. I try to get up once every hour for a little 1- to 2-minute burst of activity. It's the kind of multitasking that's good for you. Remember, your muscles don't know whether you're in the kitchen or at a fancy gym.

Here are some examples of how I exercise in my "spare time."

- Standing leg lifts as I blow-dry my hair
- Pacing or marching in place as I talk on the phone
- Two quick Pilates moves of any type between phone calls or during TV commercials
- Taking the stairs instead of the elevator at every opportunity
- "Curling" as I lift and carry grocery bags in from the car
- Squeezing my buttocks muscles and "zipping up my abs" (page 17) as I stand in line at the grocery store

The Right Shoes

To get started on my walking program, all you need is a good pair of walking shoes. Since you'll be walking purposefully, your shoes should be very comfortable. The shoes should feel flexible, allowing your feet to bend as you walk. You want good arch support to prevent your feet from rolling inward. The shoes should hug your heel while providing adequate room for your forefeet. When you try on new shoes, you should feel no pinching or rubbing, signs that the shoes don't fit well. I recommend shoes designed specifically for walking.

Proper Form

As you walk, pay attention to form. Keep your feet hip-width apart, your toes pointed straight ahead, your arms bent at 90-degree angles with your elbows held closely at your sides, your chest up and out, and your shoulders down and back. Keep your abs engaged, just as you would for Pilates practice. With each stride, plant your heel on the ground and roll through to the ball of your foot, then push off with your toes. Squeeze your buttocks as if you were trying to hold a dime between them. For maximum calorie burn, really pump those arms.

Intervals Are the Key

Walking is an excellent workout, but if you walk the same route every day at the same speed for 8 to 12 weeks, your body will start to plateau. That is, your muscles become more efficient at that pace, and you lose some of the conditioning effects. But starting from week 1, I recommend intervals—short burns of faster walking or jogging—to prevent plateaus and to jump-start your metabolism. Intervals not only will give your body a constant challenge but also will boost your metabolism and keep you motivated, helping you to stick to your routine. In each week of the 3-Week Total Body Makeover, I'll give you specific walking interval goals to strive for. If you're a beginner, you may need to work up to the amount suggested. Instead of 20 to 30 minutes total, start with just 10 minutes and work up to 20 to 30, then add in the specific workout suggested.

"For great legs, form a habit of walking wherever you can."

My In-Home Cardio Routine

If you prefer to exercise at home (so you don't have to drive anywhere or get a babysitter) or if you need to stay indoors because of bad weather, try my in-home cardio routine. Alternate between the following moves, doing each move for 2 to 3 minutes so that the routine continues for 20 to 30 minutes.

If you haven't exercised in more than a year, you may not be able to last the entire 20 to 30 minutes at first. That's okay. Start at a level you can maintain and then slowly add a few minutes at a time during each session.

I suggest in-home cardio 2 days a week and walking the other 2 days. The variety will keep you motivated as well as provide a different workout for your muscles. Remember, it's always great to change it up and "surprise" your muscles, boosting your metabolism.

1. Marching or running in place. Get those knees up high and pump those arms. Continue for 5 minutes, to warm up.

2. Crossovers. From a standing position with your hands behind your head, raise your left knee to your right elbow, lower it, then raise your right knee to your left elbow. Repeat for 2 to 3 minutes. (This is great for your waistline, too!)

3. Kicks. From a standing position with your fists at chest level (to block your imaginary opponent), lift your left knee to your waist and then kick your lower leg forward to extend your leg. Imagine kicking someone in the stomach. Tighten your abs as you do so. Lower and repeat with the other leg. Continue, switching legs, for 2 to 3 minutes. (Called front kicks in kickboxing, they're great for your legs.)

(continued on page 246)

Other Great Cardio
Workouts

Here I've listed some of the best cardio activities you can do. I like to mix and match cardio exercises, for variety. For example, some days I prefer to walk or jog. Other days I mix it up and do my *Ultimate Fat Burner* video. Choose what works best for you! The more varied your cardio routine, the more likely you'll stick with it.

As with my in-home cardio routine, start the activity that you select slowly and gradually increase the intensity and duration. If you haven't exercised in more than a year, start with 5 to 10 minutes of activity and slowly work your way up to 20 to 30 minutes in duration.

Jogging or running.
If you've been walking for some time, jogging (defined as running for 7 mph or slower) can provide a nice goal. If you've been jogging, you may want to step it up to running (faster than 7 mph). Because they raise your heart rate higher than walking does, jogging and running burn more calories per time spent than walking, making either one a wonderful fat-burning workout. Jogging and running place a lot of stress on your joints, however, and aren't good choices for those who have joint or back pain or who are seriously overweight.

Swimming and water aerobics.
If you have arthritis, bad knees, back problems, or any type of pain in general, pool workouts are ideal. Water supports the weight of your body, making you weightless and allowing you to move pain-free.

Bike riding.
Whether spinning or cycling on a stationary bike, road bike, or mountain bike, cycling provides a great calorie-burning workout. If you have a bad back or are overweight, try a recumbent bike, which allows you to lean back and relax your lower back as you cycle.

Jumping rope. This is an efficient but very challenging calorie-burning workout. It's perfect for people who can't exercise outdoors because of the weather or safety concerns and who have space to exercise indoors. If you have trouble coordinating your arms with your feet, just start by jumping without the rope and then add the rope later. For variety, try doing jumping jacks, small jumps, large jumps, and jogging with the rope.

Stairclimbers, steppers, elliptical machines, rowing machines, and other cardio equipment. Many people find working out on exercise machines very motivating. You can distract yourself by watching television as you climb stairs on the stepper, walk on the treadmill, or row on the rowing machine. Since working on any one of these machines for 30 minutes at a stretch can be tedious, mix it up by starting with 10 minutes on the stepper, then do 10 minutes on the treadmill, and 10 minutes on the rowing machine or elliptical trainer. (Unless you have the means to acquire all this equipment at home, you will probably go to a gym for this type of workout.)

Exercise videos or television workouts. I recommend videos and my televised fitness shows for people who are energized and motivated by music. Do you find yourself tapping your foot or moving your shoulders whenever a favorite song comes on the radio? Then a video set to music is probably for you. Plus, you can exercise in the privacy of your own home and don't have to drive anywhere. (If you like my in-home cardio workout, you might like to try one of my exercise videos, such as *Ultimate Fat Burner*.)

4. Punches. Stand with your knees bent and punch forward, as if you were trying to punch an imaginary opponent in the chin. Release and repeat with the other arm. Continue for 2 to 3 minutes. (Think "boxing"—punches are great for toned arms.)

5. Jump rope. If you can't continuously jump rope without getting tangled, use an imaginary rope at first, moving your body as if you were doing the real thing. Then try skipping real rope. Once you master skipping rope, try a few moves for variety such as touching your heels on the floor in front of you, jogging, or skipping like a boxer as you jump. Continue for 2 to 3 minutes. (This is great for the whole body.)

6. Jump squats. Stand with your feet together and arms at your sides. Move back into a squat as if you were sitting in a chair, keeping your abs pulled in and up. Spring up into the air, land, and repeat. Bend your knees as you land to minimize impact. Try to continue for 2 to 3 minutes. (This move is challenging. Do the best you can—it's great for the rear end!)

7. Waist twists. Pretend you're downhill skiing. With your feet together, lightly jump and pivot your knees and toes to the right as you simultaneously raise your right elbow out to the right at shoulder height and extend your left arm straight out to the left. Without lowering your arms, repeat the move in the opposite direction. Continue for 2 to 3 minutes. (I call this my "lower-body fat blast.")

8. Jack-in-the-box. With your feet together, squat as if you were sitting in a chair, then jump up and spread your feet and hands out so that your legs and arms both make an X (like a jumping jack). Position your feet together and repeat for 2 to 3 minutes. (This is also great for your inner and outer thighs!)

My Positive-Thinking PROGRAM

The thoughts in your head play a huge role in how well you stick with your 3-Week Total Body Makeover. Your mental outlook affects your energy, your enthusiasm, and your courage to try new foods, new exercises, and new habits. That's why I've included a Positive-Thinking Program in the 3-Week Total Body Makeover.

If you embark on a Pilates program without engaging your mind, you'll miss out on the relaxation, centering, focusing, and rejuvenation effects of Pilates. In Pilates, mental and physical fitness go hand in hand. Just thinking "Yes, I can do this" can help you to successfully tackle a tough Pilates pose such as a T-stand or a teaser. That can carry over to your outlook on life in general. An optimistic outlook can awaken you to new possibilities if you were previously sabotaged by self-doubt and negativity. For example, you'll find yourself tackling your career or your parenting skills with more confidence. This "I can" attitude will help you with all aspects of your life, even your relationships.

That's what makes this a comprehensive, total mind-body fitness plan. I've included some of my favorite positive-thinking tips to help you make over your mind as you make over your body.

But I also want you to do some "inner" work right now so that you start your makeover with confidence, enthusiasm, and vigor.

Make practicing Pilates your priority. Think of it as your escape, as time just for you, as your solitude among the craziness of life. For the next 3 weeks, this may take a little effort on your part. After that, your fitness routine will be habitual, and it won't take as much of a mental struggle to stick with it. In fact, you'll find yourself looking forward to your routines.

List all your exercise obstacles, with strategies for what you can do to overcome them. The number one excuse I hear for not exercising is "I don't have time." You have 10 minutes a day to improve your body, don't you? If long hours on the job keep you from exercising, then exercise at work. Walk during your lunch break, for example. While waiting for that important phone call, do Pilates exercises on the floor in your office; they'll not only tone your body but also clear your mind and help you focus! If you're at home and can't get to a gym because you don't have a babysitter, don't fret. You can do Pilates quickly at home. All you need is 4 feet of floor space. If you're open-minded and creative enough, you'll find a solution to every exercise obstacle.

Excuse-proof your brain. During the next 3 weeks, if you find yourself making excuses—telling yourself that you're going to skip just this once—remind yourself of all the reasons you started this program. Remind yourself of all the benefits you'll receive—like a longer, leaner body. Remind yourself how good you'll feel. Finally, remind yourself that every Pilates session can boost your mood, zap stress, and flush out toxins. Those days when you feel you most want to skip your routine are usually the days that you most need Pilates.

Be kind to yourself. To become more aware of your negative thoughts, try these exercises.

1. Replace judgmental words such as *klutz*, *weakling*, or *fat* with positive words such as *courage*, *challenge*, and even simply *I can*. Don't label yourself as lazy or fat—labels you'd never use to describe a friend.

2. Congratulate yourself on your devotion, discipline, and courage to try something new.

3. Accept yourself for improving the body that God gave you. Respect yourself.

Give 100 percent to Pilates in each session, but don't try to be perfect. You may sometimes feel unbalanced. You may not be able to fully extend in every Pilates move. You can't ask any more of yourself. Perfect doesn't make your practice. Rather, practice makes perfect. If you give it all you've got for 20 to 30 minutes of exercise, you will reap the benefits!

Week 1: Give Your Smile Regular Workouts

To reshape your mental outlook week by week, try the following positive-thinking techniques. Keep track of these exercises in Your Personal 3-Week Makeover Diary at the end of this program.

Days 1 and 2. When you get out of bed, go to the mirror, look at your reflection, smile, and say out loud: "I am worth it." You may feel a little silly doing so, but believe me, those simple words pack a powerful punch. The more you say it in your mind, the more you'll feel convinced. You truly are worth it!

Days 3 through 7. Continue the first exercise and take it a step further: Wear a smile wherever you go. Every time you walk through a door—whether it's to a coworker's office, your child's day-care center, or your own house—put that smile on your face and tell yourself that

Denise-eology . . .

"Enthusiasm breeds enthusiasm. Today, be the most enthusiastic person you know today."

"Why am I working out?
For my body, for my mind,
for my health, and to feel better!"

you are worth it. You'll be amazed at how easily that smile and positive attitude can affect the way people treat you, as well as the way you feel about yourself and your life! Smile, you're looking great!

Week 2: Count Your Blessings

Work on focusing on the right things—what you have to be grateful for—and avoid focusing on the wrong things—what you think you have to feel angry, sad, or frustrated about.

Days 1 through 7. Each night before you go to bed, write down five blessings. That's right—literally count your blessings. For example, I feel blessed by my two beautiful daughters, by my supportive husband, by my wonderful family and friendships, and by my fulfilling career. Finally, I remind myself every day of the wonderful gift of life.

What are your blessings? Reminding yourself each day of all the things you have to feel thankful for will help you push out those clouds of negativity and replace them with rays of hope.

Week 3: Seek Out Positive Messages

This week, I want you to start searching for messages that apply to your life in a positive way. Once you start paying attention, you'll be surprised how many positive messages you'll notice coming from everywhere—books, magazines, and even from bumper stickers.

Days 1 through 7. Find yourself an inspirational aid. Use the Denise-eology quotes sprinkled throughout this section as your inspiration. Or go to a bookstore and page through some books on poetry, quotations, or inspiring thoughts. Or subscribe to an inspiring magazine. Once you find your inspirational tool, set aside a few minutes each day to think about how the messages apply to your life.

Take note of the messages on marquees outside of churches. Regardless of your belief system or denomination, they nearly always display an interesting quote or thought. Finally, focus on the positive stories that people tell you. Once you start searching out positive messages, you'll find that there truly is more good than bad in this world.

Denise-eology . . .

"Delete the negative clutter
from your head and
put positive thoughts
in its place."

Your
3-WEEK
Pilates
PROGRAM

For the following 3 weeks, you'll practice Pilates three times a week—on Mondays, Wednesdays, and Fridays, for example. Do the moves listed in the order in which they're numbered, referring to the photo sequences and captions on the pages noted for detailed directions and pointers.

After each Pilates session, I offer two yoga cooldown stretches to help you stretch your muscles and further focus your mind. You can also use these stretches as a cooldown after your cardio routine. To fully stretch each muscle, hold each stretch for 20 to 30 seconds. I've added a Pilates Pointer of the Week to help you master the moves and stay focused and positive.

And remember: Three days a week is the minimum amount of Pilates that you need to make over your body and maintain your results. Because Pilates gently conditions your body, however, you can do Pilates as often as every day if you'd like. I personally do a 10- to 30-minute Pilates session at least 3 days a week, but some weeks I do it just about every day.

Each Food Tip of the Week is intended to help you follow the strategies and menu makeovers in My Eating Plan. And each Walk of the Week gives you a sample cardio workout if walking is your cardio exercise of choice.

As you progress through this makeover, use the 21-day diary on page 277 to keep track of your personal progress. The diary puts it all together, helping you to keep track of what you eat every day, when you do your Pilates sessions and cardio workouts, and how you feel physically and mentally as you progress.

After just 10 Pilates sessions, you'll see and feel a difference. You'll feel aware of your core abdominal muscles in your everyday life. You'll stand and sit taller. You'll feel as if you have more space between each vertebra. Your joints will feel more supple. You'll have more energy. You'll look taller and leaner. And you'll feel fit, toned, and flexible from your head to your toes.

After 3 weeks on this program, you can continue with the routines called for in week 3, or you can move on to any of the other routines in this book. I highly recommend that you mix and match routines depending on your personal goals, time constraints, and focus for any particular day. For example, on a Monday you can do the Complete Pilates Program in part 2. On a Wednesday you might try one or two of the mini-routines in part 3, and on a Friday you might try a day from week 3 of this makeover program.

Let's begin!

Week 1: Getting Started

As you start your Pilates exercises, focus on your alignment, breathing, and body positioning. If you can't do everything at once—say, matching your breathing to the movement—just focus on learning the movements. Your breathing will come.

Go slowly, checking your posture and paying attention to how your body feels in each move. You may feel awkward. That's okay. Your body must go through the motions of Pilates before those motions feel normal. Know that by next week, you'll feel a little more coordinated and balanced.

Pilates Pointer of the Week: Move through the Pilates postures without judgment. Don't think negative thoughts such as "I'll never get this." Simply trying will help you improve. Congratulate yourself for getting started, for attempting something new.

Walk of the Week: Warm up by walking for 5 minutes at your regular pace. Then begin the intervals: Speed up for 1 minute, and then bring it down a notch for 4 minutes at your normal pace. (One segment equals 1 minute at a faster pace and 4 minutes at your normal pace.) Keep alternating until you've completed four segments (20 minutes of interval walking total). At the end of your intervals, walk more slowly for 5 minutes to cool down. Do this walking workout three or four times in week 1. If you select some other form of cardio, such as swimming or biking, simulate these workout intervals by alternating the same amount of faster and slower segments.

Food Tip of the Week: Never skip breakfast, truly the most important meal of the day. Breakfast fuels your mind and body for the day ahead. If you're not a breakfast eater, start with a small, quick breakfast food this week, such as eating a small container of yogurt or a bowl of cereal. You'll be amazed at how something so simple can energize your Pilates practice as well as keep you from overeating during the rest of the day.

Denise-eology . . .

"Take a minute to sit down and make a list of things you like about yourself. For instance, you have a great smile, you have toned arms, or you're a great friend."

Session 1

1

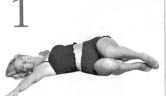

Warmup Stretch with Knee Sway (page 36)

2

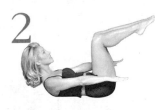

Beginner Hundred (page 44)

3

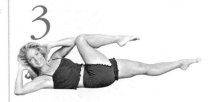

Crisscross (page 78)

4

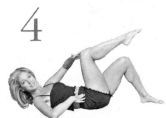

One-Leg Lift (page 42)

5

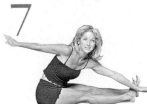

Single-Leg Teaser (page 95)

6

T-Stand (page 86)

7

The Saw (page 80)

8

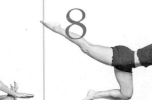

Back Strengthener (page 58)

9

Chest Expansion (page 111)

10

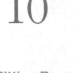

Sitting Pose Sequence (page 148)

YOGA COOLDOWN →

11 Forward Bend with Twist

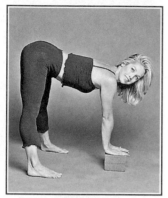 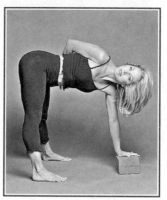

A. Spread your feet slightly wider than hip width apart. Pull your abs toward your spine and bend forward from the waist, keeping your back flat. If you can do it comfortably, place your palms on the floor. If you can't, use a block or a stack of books as a prop, as shown.

B. Keeping your hips level, support your body weight with your left arm and rotate to the right, initiating the movement with your lower spine. Place your right arm behind your back, to help maintain proper posture. Open your chest and breathe deeply. Switch sides.

12 Eagle

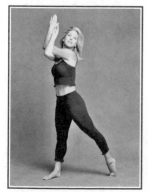

Stand with your feet under your hips, your belly button pressed toward your spine, your shoulders down, and your chest open. Put your body weight into your right foot and step back with your left, using the toes of your left foot for balance. Keep your abs flat and your hips level. Bend your left arm and bring your left elbow in front of your sternum (breastbone) with the fingers of your left hand pointing toward the ceiling. Thread your right arm under your left elbow and then up, as shown, so that the top of your right forearm is touching the top of your left forearm. If you can, try to touch your left and right palms together, feeling a deep stretch between your shoulder blades, opening your upper back muscles and releasing tension between the shoulder blades. Press forward with your elbows to deepen the stretch. Switch arms.

Session 2

1

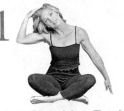

Neck-Shoulder-Back
Relaxer (page 188)

2

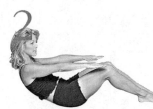

Roll-Ups Preparation
(page 46)

3

Bridge (page 70)

4

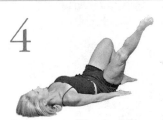

Beginner Single-Leg
Ciroles (page 49)

5

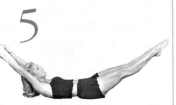

Double-Leg Tummy Tuck
(page 183)

6

Seated Spinal Twist
(page 89)

7

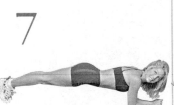

Low Hover (page 181)

8

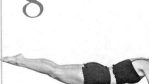

Leg Raise (page 82)

9

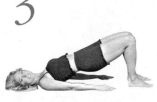

Chest Lift
(page 112)

10

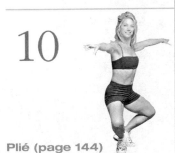

Plié (page 144)

YOGA COOLDOWN →

11 Modified Downward Facing Dog with Chair

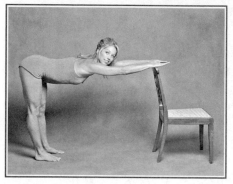

Stand 2 to 3 feet behind a chair. Reach your arms overhead and bend forward from your hips, controlling your forward movement with the strength of your abs. Rest your hands on the back of the chair, as shown. If your feet are in front of your hips, move them back. Then breathe deeply as you stretch back through your tailbone.

12 Modified Dancer's Pose

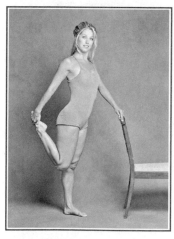

Stand a foot away from a chair. Place your body weight onto your left foot. Bend your right knee, bringing your right foot toward your buttocks. Grasp your right ankle with your right hand, as shown. Pull your abs to your spine and focus on extending your right knee down, toward the floor. Breathe deeply as your thigh relaxes. Repeat with the other leg.

Session 3

1

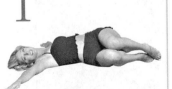

Warmup Stretch with Knee Sway (page 36)

2

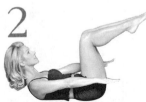

Beginner Hundred (page 44)

3

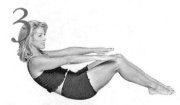

Roll-Ups Preparation (page 46)

4

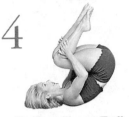

Rolling like a Ball (page 50)

5

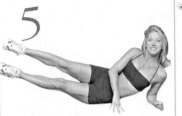

Leg Beats (page 153)

6

Bun Lifter (page 150)

7

Swimming (page 84)

8

Leg Pull Front (page 101)

9

Alternating Arms Scissors (page 113)

10

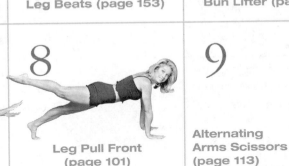

Leg Extension Sequence (page 146)

YOGA COOLDOWN →

11 Hamstring Stretch Sequence

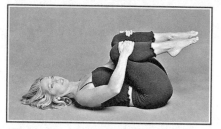

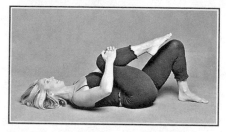

A. Lie on your back with your knees gently pulled in toward your chest and your hands resting just below your knees. Press your belly button toward your spine.

B. Lower your feet to the floor. Bring your right knee in toward your chest, as shown, feeling a stretch along the back of your right leg and buttock.

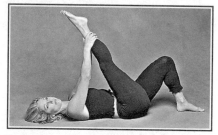

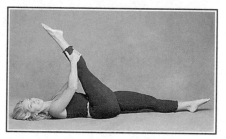

C. Straighten your right leg and use your hands on your calf to gently increase the stretch, breathing deeply.

D. If you can, straighten your left leg against the floor. Hold and then repeat on the other side.

12 Lateral Spiral Stretch

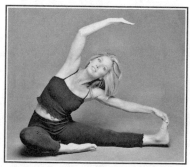

Sit with your legs extended in front of you. Bend your right knee and bring your right foot in close to your left inner thigh. Rotate your body so that your chest is facing your right knee. Bend from your waist toward your left foot, sliding your left hand along your left leg, reaching for your toes. Bring your right arm overhead, as shown, feeling a deep stretch along the right side of your body. Then switch sides.

Week 2: Progress Gradually

During week 1, you started with Pilates exercises that strengthened your core and stretched out your entire body. In week 2, you will progress gradually. Some of the exercises will take you up a level, to intermediate moves. The upper body exercises for this week incorporate light weights, so have a set of dumbbells handy. If you don't have dumbbells, you can also use 1-liter water bottles filled with water. If you feel that some of the moves are still too difficult, that's okay. Just modify them as described in my Complete Pilates Program on page 63.

Pilates Pointer of the Week: Now that you're familiar with many of the Pilates moves, try to move with your breath. Try to move as you exhale and inhale, matching your movement to your breathing. This will make your Pilates session more meditative, soothing away stress and tension.

Walk of the Week: Warm up for 5 minutes at your regular pace. Then speed up for 2 minutes, and then recover for 3 minutes at your normal pace. Keep alternating 2 minutes at a faster pace with 3 minutes at your normal pace until you've completed four segments. (One segment equals 2 minutes at a faster pace plus 3 minutes at a normal pace.) At the end of your intervals, walk slowly for 5 minutes to cool down. Do this walking workout three or four times this week. If you'd rather do some other form of cardio, you can simulate this interval workout by alternating the same period of faster and slower segments. Remember, intervals are a great way to rev up your metabolism.

Food Tip of the Week: Brush your teeth mentally and physically after dinner. It's a simple symbol that means you're done for the night. Plus, toothpaste alters the taste of anything you eat. I like to brush my teeth right after dinner. That way I won't pig out later in the evening.

Session 1

1
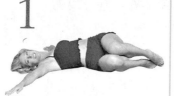
Warmup Stretch with Knee Sway (page 36)

2
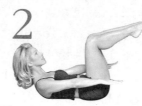
The Hundred (page 66) —Do half with knees bent.

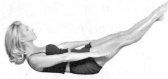
—Do half with legs straight.

3
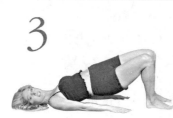
Bridge (page 70)

4

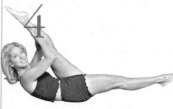
Single Straight-Leg Stretch (page 77)

5
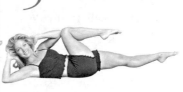
Crisscross (page 78)

6
Superman (page 83)

7
T-Stand with Twist (page 87)

8
Side Leg Lift—More Challenging (page 90)

9
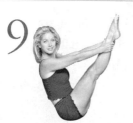
Teaser (page 96)

10
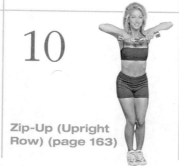
Zip-Up (Upright Row) (page 163)

YOGA COOLDOWN →

11 Lateral Stretch

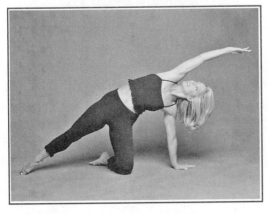

Sit with your legs extended. Bend your left knee and bring your left foot next to your inner right thigh. Sweep your right arm overhead as you inhale and raise yourself onto your left knee, as shown. Support your body weight evenly between your left hand and knee and your right foot. Reach through your right fingers, feeling a deep stretch from your outer thigh all the way to your fingertips. Repeat on the other side.

12 Warrior

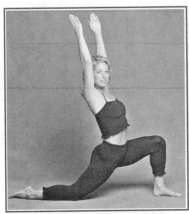

From a standing position, take a large step forward with your left leg, bending your left knee at a 90-degree angle and extending your right leg back, allowing your right shin to rest on the floor, if you can. Sink into the pose, trying to keep both hipbones facing forward. You should feel the work in your left buttocks and hamstrings. Extend through your torso, flatten your abs toward your spine, and reach your arms overhead, as shown, feeling a deep stretch through the front of your body, especially your hip flexors. Repeat on the other side.

Session 2

1
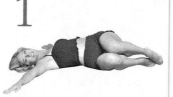

Warmup Stretch with Knee Sway (page 36)

2
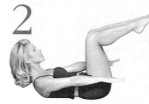 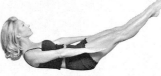

The Hundred (page 66)
—Do half with knees bent.

—Do half with legs straight.

3
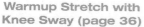
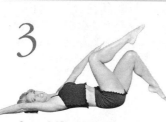

Leg Lift with Reach (page 52)

4

The Roll-Up (page 68)

5

Double-Leg Stretch (page 76)

6
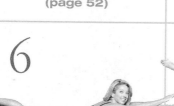

Swimming (page 84)

7
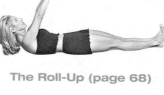

Side Leg Circles—More Challenging (page 91)

8

Leg Pull Back (page 100)

9
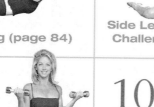

Strong Man (page 164)

10
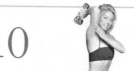 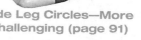 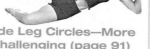

Triceps Toner (page 169)

YOGA COOLDOWN →

11 Neck-Shoulder-Back Relaxer

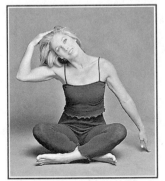 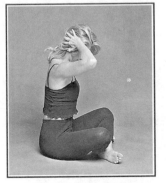 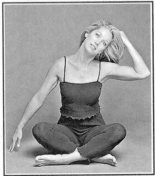

A. Sit comfortably with your legs crossed. Sit tall and bring your weight onto your "sit bones," engage your abs, and lengthen through the crown of your head. Place your left hand on the floor. Exhale and lower your right ear toward your right shoulder, as shown. Gently use your right fingers to increase the stretch in your neck.

B. Inhale and roll your head forward, bringing your chin close to your upper chest. Gently use the fingers of both hands to increase the stretch to the back of your neck and shoulders.

C. Exhale and roll your head to the left. Place your right hand on the floor. Gently use the fingers of your left hand to increase the stretch to the side of your neck.

12 Open Leg Stretch

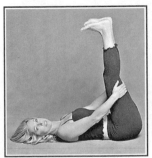

A. Lie on your back with your legs raised and extended to a 90-degree angle with your torso. To straighten your legs, press your heels toward the ceiling, as shown.

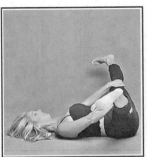

B. Slowly lower your legs and extend them to the sides so that they form a V, with your toes angled toward the floor. This is great for leg circulation.

Session 3

1
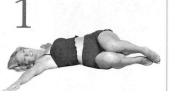
Warmup Stretch with
Knee Sway (page 36)

2
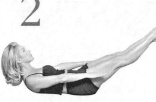
The Hundred (page 67)

3
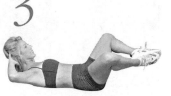
The Frog (page 174)

4
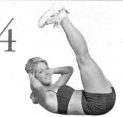
Double-Leg Lift
(page 175)

5
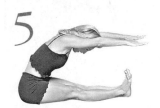
Spine Stretch Forward
(page 79)

6
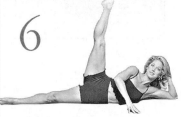
Side Leg Lift—More
Challenging (page 90)

7
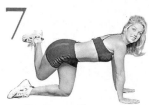
Bottom Firmer
Sequence (page 151)

8
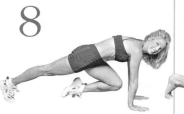
Plank (page 179)

9
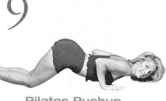
Pilates Pushup
(page 103)

10
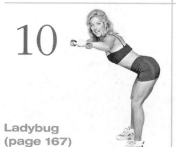
Ladybug
(page 167)

YOGA COOLDOWN →

11 Cat Stretch

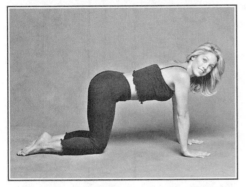

A. Get on all fours with your hands under your shoulders and knees under your hips. Press your abs toward your spine.

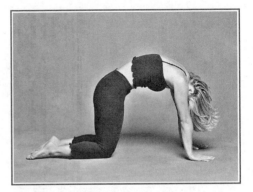

B. Exhale as you engage your abs and draw your navel in toward your spine even further, curling your hipbones down and forming a C shape with your spine.

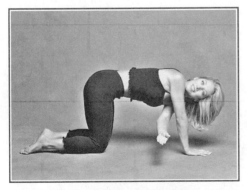

C. Return your spine to the flat position. Inhale as you thread your extended left arm under your body to the right, as shown, feeling a nice stretch along the left side of your back. Return your left hand to the floor and repeat with your right arm.

Denise-eology . . .
"Food isn't the enemy. Sitting still is."

12 Total Back Relaxer

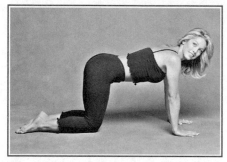

A. Kneel on your hands and knees, with your abs lifted and your back flat. Your hands should be directly under your shoulders and your knees directly under your hips, with the tops of your feet flat on the floor.

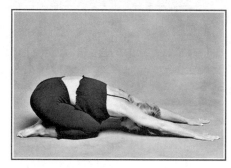

B. From your abs, move your hips back, bringing your buttocks onto your heels and resting your belly on your thighs. Keep your hands firmly in position throughout the move. Take three deep, cleansing breaths, then relax.

Week 3: Feel the Difference

Keep it up—you're doing great! This week you will start to see and *feel* a difference! Your posture is improving, your abs are stronger, and your arms and legs are firmer.

This week's routine again steps up the level of difficulty. Try all of the suggested Pilates exercises. If a few are beyond your ability right now, just do the basic version of the exercise shown in the Beginner Pilates Program and avoid moves marked "more challenging" from the Complete Pilates Program. No matter what level of effort you choose, you will still be toning that particular muscle or group of muscles.

Pilates is very fluid, so take your time. This is not a competition. It is a gradual way to progress and challenge your body. The three different workouts in week 3 are some of the advanced versions in Pilates. Just do your best and always give 110 percent effort.

Pilates Pointer of the Week: Before you know it, people will be asking you the secret to your energy and your staying calm and clearheaded. Before your practice, take a deep breath and let it out with a sigh, releasing everything that's on your mind, letting it all go. Notice where your mind is as you move. Listen deeply to your body. What is it telling you today?

Stay mindful during your workout. Try not to allow yourself to think of work or daily responsibilities. This is your time to just be. Focus inward on your breath, your muscles, your alignment, your body. This inward focus will leave you feeling refreshed, calm, and rejuvenated after your routine. Try to carry that calmness with you all day long, being the calm in everyone else's daily storm of life. Each day, make this sense of serenity last a little longer.

Walk of the Week: Warm up for 5 minutes at your regular pace. Speed up for 3 minutes, then recover for 2 minutes by walking at your normal pace. (One segment equals 3 minutes at a faster pace and 2 minutes at your normal pace.) Keep alternating 3 minutes at a faster pace with 2 minutes at your regular pace until you've completed four segments. At the end of your intervals, walk for 5 minutes to cool down. Do this 30-minute walk workout three or four times this week. If you'd rather do some other form of cardio, you can adapt this workout by alternating the same amount of faster and slower segments.

Food Tip of the Week: An easy way to improve your diet is by eating whole fruit rather than drinking juice. For example, eating an orange or grapefruit rather than drinking the juice gives you extra fiber, which prevents heart disease and helps you feel satiated so that you'll feel less inclined to overeat. Eating a piece of fruit also takes longer than drinking a glass of juice, so you feel more mentally satisfied afterward.

Session 1

1

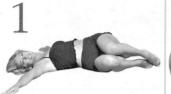

Warmup Stretch with Knee Sway (page 36)

2

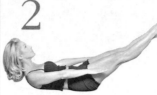

The Hundred (page 67) —Do half with toes pointed.

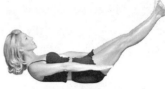

—Do half with toes turned out.

3

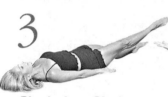

Single-Leg Circles— More Challenging (page 73)

4

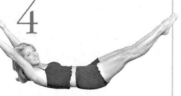

Double-Leg Stretch (page 76)

5

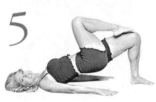

Bridge—More Challenging (page 71)

6

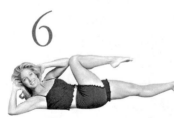

Crisscross (page 78)

7

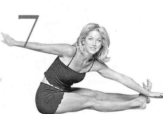

The Saw (page 80)

8

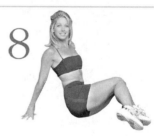

Can-Can (page 177)

9

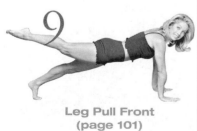

Leg Pull Front (page 101)

10

Double-Arm Row (page 170)

YOGA COOLDOWN →

11 Foot, Ankle, and Leg Stretch

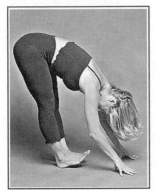

A. Begin in a forward bend position, resting your hands on the floor for balance. Rock your body weight back onto your heels, as shown, and lift the balls of your feet up, stretching your ankles, calves, and Achilles tendons.

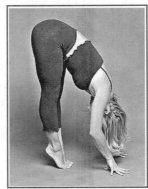

B. Adjust your body weight, bringing it forward onto the balls of your feet and raising your heels. Feel a stretch in your shins and along the tops of your feet.

12 Hip Circles

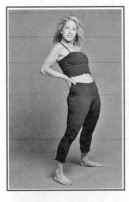

A. Stand with your feet slightly wider than hip width apart. Tighten your abs and place your hands along your lower back. Keeping your abs pressed flat, bring your lower torso forward, as shown, feeling a stretch along your lower abs.

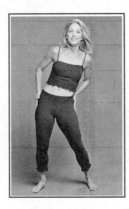

B. Bring your hips to the right, feeling a stretch along the right side of your hips and waist. Continue circling your hips until you've made a complete revolution. Then reverse direction.

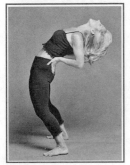

C. Now, with your hips pressed forward, bend slightly back, feeling a deep stretch along the front of your torso. Make sure to elongate your spine and squeeze your buttocks to eliminate any pinching in your back. Also, keep those abs engaged.

Session 2

1
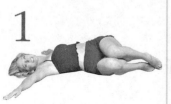

Warmup Stretch with Knee Sway (page 36)

2
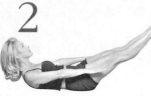

The Hundred (page 67)
—Do half with toes pointed.

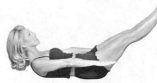

—Do half with toes turned out.

3
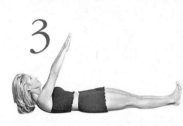

The Roll-Up (page 68)

4
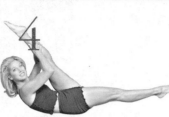

Single Straight-Leg Stretch (page 77)

5
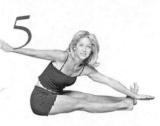

The Saw (page 80)

6
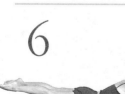

Superman (page 83)

7
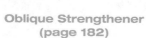

Oblique Strengthener (page 182)

8
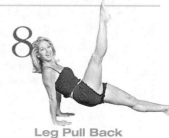

Leg Pull Back (page 100)

9
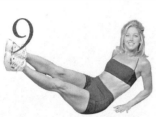

Can-Can Extension (page 178)

10

Overhead Press (page 171)

YOGA COOLDOWN →

11 Downward Facing Dog with Leg Stretch

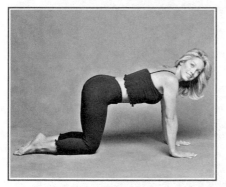

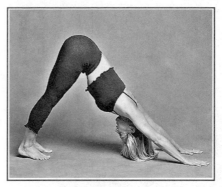

A. From all fours with your hands under your shoulders and your knees under your hips, pull your abs toward your spine as you exhale and press back through your palms and bring your buttocks close to your heels.

B. Bring the balls of your feet onto the floor and, keeping your abs engaged, inhale and raise your tailbone toward the ceiling, as shown. Eventually, you'll want to press your heels toward the floor. If you aren't yet flexible enough to do that, start with your knees slightly bent, concentrating on pressing your tailbone to the sky and scooping your abs in toward your spine. Slowly try to straighten your legs.

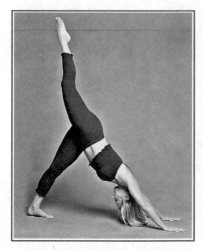

C. Once you can lower your heels close to the floor without losing the scoop in your abs or your long, flat back, shift your body weight onto your left foot and, while keeping your hips level, raise your right leg up, as shown. At first you may not be able to fully extend your right leg. That's fine. Allow your calf to stretch as you concentrate on keeping your abs pressed against your spine and your hips level. Visualize bringing your right hipbone down and forward while pushing your left hipbone back and up. Take three deep, cleansing breaths and then switch legs. Now come back to downward facing dog with both legs together and then relax.

12 Mermaid

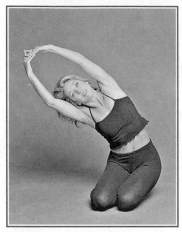

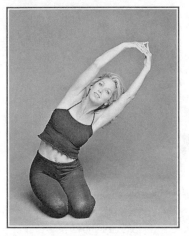

A. Kneel with your heels by your buttocks. Lengthen your spine by lifting the crown of your head upward and pressing down through your tailbone. Flatten your abs toward your spine. Reach both arms overhead and grasp your fingers together. Reach your arms and torso to the right, as shown, feeling the stretch along the left side of your body.

B. Inhale as you return to center and exhale as you reach to the left, feeling the stretch along the right side of your body.

Session 3

1
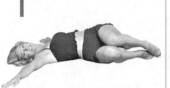
Warmup Stretch with Knee Sway (page 36)

2
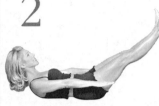
The Hundred (page 67)

3
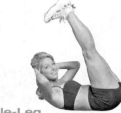
Double-Leg Lift (page 175)

4
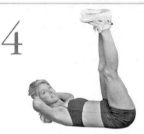
Corkscrew (page 176)

5
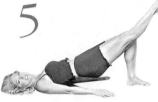
Bridge—More Challenging (page 71)

6
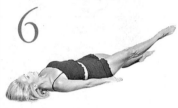
Single-Leg Circles—More Challenging (page 73)

7
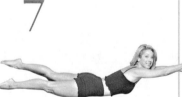
Swimming (page 84)

8
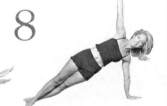
Advanced T-Stand—Even More Challenging (page 88)

9
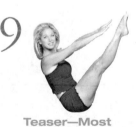
Teaser—Most Challenging (page 97)

10
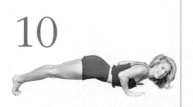
Pilates Pushup—More Challenging (page 104)

YOGA COOLDOWN ⟶

11 Hamstring and Back Stretch

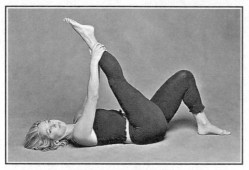

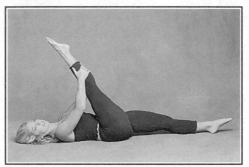

A. Lie on your back with your knees pulled gently in toward your chest. Press your belly button toward your spine. Lower your feet to the floor. Bring your right knee in toward your chest. Straighten your right leg, as shown, and use your hands on your calf to gently increase the stretch, breathing deeply.

B. If you can, straighten your left leg against the floor. Repeat on the other side.

12 Triangle

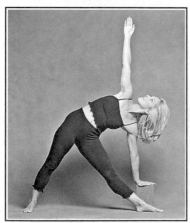

Stand with your feet in a wide angle, forming a V shape. Turn your left foot out so that your left heel is facing your right ankle. Angle your right heel out slightly. Square your hips and flatten your abs toward your spine. Reach both arms out to the sides and lengthen through the crown of your head. Press through your left hand as you move your entire torso to the left. Then lower your left hand toward the floor. Eventually, you'll want to reach the floor in front of your left foot, but if you lack the balance, strength, and flexibility, you can hold on to your calf. Open your chest toward the ceiling. Feel a deep stretch along the outside of your body. Feel your hips and chest open. Repeat on the other side.

Your PERSONAL 3-Week MAKEOVER Diary

designed the 3-Week Total Body Makeover to simplify your life. It lays out everything you need—eating strategies, menu plans, workout routines, and week-by-week tips for positive thinking. Use the diary on the following pages to keep track of your improvement. The diary provides space for you to track each element of your makeover—nutrition, Pilates sessions, cardio exercise, positive thinking, and the results you see and feel.

For the eating plan, check off the total number of food servings for the calorie level you've chosen to follow. For days when Pilates or cardio aren't scheduled, leave those sections blank. Write about your daily positive-thinking exercises and note the results you feel from the makeover in the spaces provided.

Fill in your diary each night before you go to bed, making sure to give yourself enough time to use the diary to plan for the following day.

If you want to continue beyond 3 weeks, photocopy the last page of the diary.

Day 1

MY EATING PLAN

Food	Daily Servings		
Fruits and Vegetables	1,350-Calorie Plan ☐1 ☐2 ☐3 ☐4 ☐5	1,600-Calorie Plan ☐6 ☐7	2,200-Calorie Plan ☐8 ☐9
Whole Grains	1,350- and 1,600-Calorie Plans ☐1 ☐2 ☐3 ☐4 ☐5 ☐6		2,200-Calorie Plan ☐7 ☐8 ☐9
Starch	1,350-Calorie Plan ☐1	1,600-Calorie Plan ☐2	2,200-Calorie Plan ☐3
Protein	All Plans ☐1 ☐2		
Dairy	All Plans ☐1 ☐2		
Fat	1,350-Calorie Plan ☐1 ☐2 ☐3 ☐4	1,600-Calorie Plan ☐5 ☐6	2,200-Calorie Plan ☐7 ☐8
Water	All Plans ☐1 ☐2 ☐3 ☐4 ☐5 ☐6 ☐7 ☐8		

Healthiest foods I selected today:

_____

_____

_____

How I can improve tomorrow:

_____

_____

_____

_____

_____

PILATES

☐ I did a Pilates session today.   ☐ I did my warmup and cooldown stretches.

CARDIO EXERCISE

Type of cardio I did today: _____

Minutes of cardio I did today: _____   Day of my next cardio session: _____

POSITIVE THINKING

Positive-thinking exercise I did today: _____   ☐ I made time for me today.

How I felt about myself today: _____

How I can feel even better tomorrow: _____

RESULTS

Changes I see so far today (lengthening, toning, and so forth): _____

_____

Changes I feel so far (strengthening, energy levels, mental outlook, and so forth): _____

_____

Other improvements: _____

_____

Additional thoughts: _____

_____

Day 2

MY EATING PLAN

Food	Daily Servings			Healthiest foods I selected today:

Fruits and Vegetables

1,350-Calorie Plan	1,600-Calorie Plan	2,200-Calorie Plan
☐1 ☐2 ☐3 ☐4 ☐5	☐6 ☐7	☐8 ☐9

Whole Grains

1,350- and 1,600-Calorie Plans	2,200-Calorie Plan
☐1 ☐2 ☐3 ☐4 ☐5 ☐6	☐7 ☐8 ☐9

Starch

1,350-Calorie Plan	1,600-Calorie Plan	2,200-Calorie Plan
☐1	☐2	☐3

Protein — All Plans ☐1 ☐2

Dairy — All Plans ☐1 ☐2

Fat

1,350-Calorie Plan	1,600-Calorie Plan	2,200-Calorie Plan
☐1 ☐2 ☐3 ☐4	☐5 ☐6	☐7 ☐8

Water — All Plans ☐1 ☐2 ☐3 ☐4 ☐5 ☐6 ☐7 ☐8

Healthiest foods I selected today:

_____
_____
_____
_____

How I can improve tomorrow:

_____
_____
_____
_____
_____
_____

PILATES

☐ I did a Pilates session today.　☐ I did my warmup and cooldown stretches.

CARDIO EXERCISE

Type of cardio I did today: _____

Minutes of cardio I did today: _____ Day of my next cardio session: _____

POSITIVE THINKING

Positive-thinking exercise I did today: _____ ☐ I made time for me today.

How I felt about myself today: _____

How I can feel even better tomorrow: _____

RESULTS

Changes I see so far today (lengthening, toning, and so forth): _____

_____

Changes I feel so far (strengthening, energy levels, mental outlook, and so forth): _____

_____

Other improvements: _____

_____

Additional thoughts: _____

_____

Day 3 MY EATING PLAN

Food	Daily Servings			Healthiest foods I selected today:

Fruits and Vegetables	1,350-Calorie Plan ☐1 ☐2 ☐3 ☐4 ☐5	1,600-Calorie Plan ☐6 ☐7	2,200-Calorie Plan ☐8 ☐9

Healthiest foods I selected today:

_____

_____

_____

Whole Grains	1,350- and 1,600-Calorie Plans ☐1 ☐2 ☐3 ☐4 ☐5 ☐6	2,200-Calorie Plan ☐7 ☐8 ☐9

Starch	1,350-Calorie Plan ☐1	1,600-Calorie Plan ☐2	2,200-Calorie Plan ☐3

How I can improve tomorrow:

_____

Protein	All Plans ☐1 ☐2

Dairy	All Plans ☐1 ☐2

_____

Fat	1,350-Calorie Plan ☐1 ☐2 ☐3 ☐4	1,600-Calorie Plan ☐5 ☐6	2,200-Calorie Plan ☐7 ☐8

_____

Water	All Plans ☐1 ☐2 ☐3 ☐4 ☐5 ☐6 ☐7 ☐8

_____

_____

PILATES

☐ I did a Pilates session today.   ☐ I did my warmup and cooldown stretches.

CARDIO EXERCISE

Type of cardio I did today: _____

Minutes of cardio I did today: _____ Day of my next cardio session: _____

POSITIVE THINKING

Positive-thinking exercise I did today: _____ ☐ I made time for me today.

How I felt about myself today: _____

How I can feel even better tomorrow: _____

RESULTS

Changes I see so far today (lengthening, toning, and so forth): _____

_____

Changes I feel so far (strengthening, energy levels, mental outlook, and so forth): _____

_____

Other improvements: _____

_____

Additional thoughts: _____

_____

Day 4 MY EATING PLAN

Food	Daily Servings			Healthiest foods I selected today:

Fruits and Vegetables

1,350-Calorie Plan	1,600-Calorie Plan	2,200-Calorie Plan
☐1 ☐2 ☐3 ☐4 ☐5	☐6 ☐7	☐8 ☐9

Whole Grains

1,350- and 1,600-Calorie Plans	2,200-Calorie Plan
☐1 ☐2 ☐3 ☐4 ☐5 ☐6	☐7 ☐8 ☐9

Starch

1,350-Calorie Plan	1,600-Calorie Plan	2,200-Calorie Plan
☐1	☐2	☐3

Protein All Plans ☐1 ☐2

Dairy All Plans ☐1 ☐2

How I can improve tomorrow:

_____

_____

_____

_____

Fat

1,350-Calorie Plan	1,600-Calorie Plan	2,200-Calorie Plan
☐1 ☐2 ☐3 ☐4	☐5 ☐6	☐7 ☐8

Water All Plans ☐1 ☐2 ☐3 ☐4 ☐5 ☐6 ☐7 ☐8

_____

_____

_____

PILATES

☐ I did a Pilates session today. ☐ I did my warmup and cooldown stretches.

CARDIO EXERCISE

Type of cardio I did today: _____

Minutes of cardio I did today: _____ Day of my next cardio session: _____

POSITIVE THINKING

Positive-thinking exercise I did today: _____ ☐ I made time for me today.

How I felt about myself today: _____

How I can feel even better tomorrow: _____

RESULTS

Changes I see so far today (lengthening, toning, and so forth): _____

_____

Changes I feel so far (strengthening, energy levels, mental outlook, and so forth): _____

_____

Other improvements: _____

_____

Additional thoughts: _____

_____

Day 5   MY EATING PLAN

Food	Daily Servings		

Healthiest foods I selected today:

_____
_____
_____
_____

Fruits and Vegetables

1,350-Calorie Plan	1,600-Calorie Plan	2,200-Calorie Plan
☐1 ☐2 ☐3 ☐4 ☐5	☐6 ☐7	☐8 ☐9

Whole Grains

1,350- and 1,600-Calorie Plans	2,200-Calorie Plan
☐1 ☐2 ☐3 ☐4 ☐5 ☐6	☐7 ☐8 ☐9

Starch

1,350-Calorie Plan	1,600-Calorie Plan	2,200-Calorie Plan
☐1	☐2	☐3

How I can improve tomorrow:

_____
_____
_____

Protein   All Plans ☐1 ☐2

Dairy   All Plans ☐1 ☐2

Fat

1,350-Calorie Plan	1,600-Calorie Plan	2,200-Calorie Plan
☐1 ☐2 ☐3 ☐4	☐5 ☐6	☐7 ☐8

Water   All Plans ☐1 ☐2 ☐3 ☐4 ☐5 ☐6 ☐7 ☐8

_____
_____
_____

PILATES

☐ I did a Pilates session today.   ☐ I did my warmup and cooldown stretches.

CARDIO EXERCISE

Type of cardio I did today: _____

Minutes of cardio I did today: _____ Day of my next cardio session: _____

POSITIVE THINKING

Positive-thinking exercise I did today: _____ ☐ I made time for me today.

How I felt about myself today: _____

How I can feel even better tomorrow: _____

RESULTS

Changes I see so far today (lengthening, toning, and so forth): _____
_____

Changes I feel so far (strengthening, energy levels, mental outlook, and so forth): _____
_____

Other improvements: _____
_____

Additional thoughts: _____

Day 6

MY EATING PLAN

Food	Daily Servings		
Fruits and Vegetables	1,350-Calorie Plan ☐1 ☐2 ☐3 ☐4 ☐5	1,600-Calorie Plan ☐6 ☐7	2,200-Calorie Plan ☐8 ☐9
Whole Grains	1,350- and 1,600-Calorie Plans ☐1 ☐2 ☐3 ☐4 ☐5 ☐6		2,200-Calorie Plan ☐7 ☐8 ☐9
Starch	1,350-Calorie Plan ☐1	1,600-Calorie Plan ☐2	2,200-Calorie Plan ☐3
Protein	All Plans ☐1 ☐2		
Dairy	All Plans ☐1 ☐2		
Fat	1,350-Calorie Plan ☐1 ☐2 ☐3 ☐4	1,600-Calorie Plan ☐5 ☐6	2,200-Calorie Plan ☐7 ☐8
Water	All Plans ☐1 ☐2 ☐3 ☐4 ☐5 ☐6 ☐7 ☐8		

Healthiest foods I selected today:

_____

_____

_____

How I can improve tomorrow:

_____

_____

_____

_____

_____

PILATES

☐ I did a Pilates session today.   ☐ I did my warmup and cooldown stretches.

CARDIO EXERCISE

Type of cardio I did today: _____

Minutes of cardio I did today: _____   Day of my next cardio session: _____

POSITIVE THINKING

Positive-thinking exercise I did today: _____   ☐ I made time for me today.

How I felt about myself today: _____

How I can feel even better tomorrow: _____

RESULTS

Changes I see so far today (lengthening, toning, and so forth): _____

_____

Changes I feel so far (strengthening, energy levels, mental outlook, and so forth): _____

_____

Other improvements: _____

_____

Additional thoughts: _____

_____

Day 7   MY EATING PLAN

Food	Daily Servings			Healthiest foods I selected today:

Fruits and Vegetables	1,350-Calorie Plan ☐1 ☐2 ☐3 ☐4 ☐5	1,600-Calorie Plan ☐6 ☐7	2,200-Calorie Plan ☐8 ☐9
Whole Grains	1,350- and 1,600-Calorie Plans ☐1 ☐2 ☐3 ☐4 ☐5 ☐6		2,200-Calorie Plan ☐7 ☐8 ☐9
Starch	1,350-Calorie Plan ☐1	1,600-Calorie Plan ☐2	2,200-Calorie Plan ☐3
Protein	All Plans ☐1 ☐2		
Dairy	All Plans ☐1 ☐2		
Fat	1,350-Calorie Plan ☐1 ☐2 ☐3 ☐4	1,600-Calorie Plan ☐5 ☐6	2,200-Calorie Plan ☐7 ☐8
Water	All Plans ☐1 ☐2 ☐3 ☐4 ☐5 ☐6 ☐7 ☐8		

_____
_____
_____

How I can improve tomorrow:

_____
_____
_____
_____
_____
_____

PILATES

☐ I did a Pilates session today.   ☐ I did my warmup and cooldown stretches.

CARDIO EXERCISE

Type of cardio I did today: _____

Minutes of cardio I did today: _____ Day of my next cardio session: _____

POSITIVE THINKING

Positive-thinking exercise I did today: _____ ☐ I made time for me today.

How I felt about myself today: _____

How I can feel even better tomorrow: _____

RESULTS

Changes I see so far today (lengthening, toning, and so forth): _____
_____

Changes I feel so far (strengthening, energy levels, mental outlook, and so forth): _____
_____

Other improvements: _____
_____

Additional thoughts: _____
_____

Day 8

MY EATING PLAN

Food	Daily Servings		
Fruits and Vegetables	1,350-Calorie Plan ☐1 ☐2 ☐3 ☐4 ☐5	1,600-Calorie Plan ☐6 ☐7	2,200-Calorie Plan ☐8 ☐9
Whole Grains	1,350- and 1,600-Calorie Plans ☐1 ☐2 ☐3 ☐4 ☐5 ☐6		2,200-Calorie Plan ☐7 ☐8 ☐9
Starch	1,350-Calorie Plan ☐1	1,600-Calorie Plan ☐2	2,200-Calorie Plan ☐3
Protein	All Plans ☐1 ☐2		
Dairy	All Plans ☐1 ☐2		
Fat	1,350-Calorie Plan ☐1 ☐2 ☐3 ☐4	1,600-Calorie Plan ☐5 ☐6	2,200-Calorie Plan ☐7 ☐8
Water	All Plans ☐1 ☐2 ☐3 ☐4 ☐5 ☐6 ☐7 ☐8		

Healthiest foods I selected today:

_____
_____
_____
_____

How I can improve tomorrow:

_____
_____
_____
_____
_____
_____

PILATES

☐ I did a Pilates session today.   ☐ I did my warmup and cooldown stretches.

CARDIO EXERCISE

Type of cardio I did today: _____

Minutes of cardio I did today: _____ Day of my next cardio session: _____

POSITIVE THINKING

Positive-thinking exercise I did today: _____ ☐ I made time for me today.

How I felt about myself today: _____

How I can feel even better tomorrow: _____

RESULTS

Changes I see so far today (lengthening, toning, and so forth): _____

_____

Changes I feel so far (strengthening, energy levels, mental outlook, and so forth): _____

_____

Other improvements: _____

_____

Additional thoughts: _____

_____

Day 9

MY EATING PLAN

Food	Daily Servings			Healthiest foods I selected today:
Fruits and Vegetables	1,350-Calorie Plan ☐1 ☐2 ☐3 ☐4 ☐5	1,600-Calorie Plan ☐6 ☐7	2,200-Calorie Plan ☐8 ☐9	_____ _____
Whole Grains	1,350- and 1,600-Calorie Plans ☐1 ☐2 ☐3 ☐4 ☐5 ☐6		2,200-Calorie Plan ☐7 ☐8 ☐9	_____ _____
Starch	1,350-Calorie Plan ☐1	1,600-Calorie Plan ☐2	2,200-Calorie Plan ☐3	How I can improve tomorrow:
Protein	All Plans ☐1 ☐2			_____
Dairy	All Plans ☐1 ☐2			_____
Fat	1,350-Calorie Plan ☐1 ☐2 ☐3 ☐4	1,600-Calorie Plan ☐5 ☐6	2,200-Calorie Plan ☐7 ☐8	_____ _____
Water	All Plans ☐1 ☐2 ☐3 ☐4 ☐5 ☐6 ☐7 ☐8			_____ _____

PILOTES

PILATES

☐ I did a Pilates session today.   ☐ I did my warmup and cooldown stretches.

CARDIO EXERCISE

Type of cardio I did today: _____

Minutes of cardio I did today: _____ Day of my next cardio session: _____

POSITIVE THINKING

Positive-thinking exercise I did today: _____ ☐ I made time for me today.

How I felt about myself today: _____

How I can feel even better tomorrow: _____

RESULTS

Changes I see so far today (lengthening, toning, and so forth): _____

_____

Changes I feel so far (strengthening, energy levels, mental outlook, and so forth): _____

_____

Other improvements: _____

_____

Additional thoughts: _____

_____

Day 10 MY EATING PLAN

Food	Daily Servings			Healthiest foods I selected today:

| **Fruits and Vegetables** | 1,350-Calorie Plan ☐1 ☐2 ☐3 ☐4 ☐5 | 1,600-Calorie Plan ☐6 ☐7 | 2,200-Calorie Plan ☐8 ☐9 |

_____

_____

| **Whole Grains** | 1,350- and 1,600-Calorie Plans ☐1 ☐2 ☐3 ☐4 ☐5 ☐6 | 2,200-Calorie Plan ☐7 ☐8 ☐9 |

_____

| **Starch** | 1,350-Calorie Plan ☐1 | 1,600-Calorie Plan ☐2 | 2,200-Calorie Plan ☐3 |

How I can improve tomorrow:

| **Protein** | All Plans ☐1 ☐2 |

_____

| **Dairy** | All Plans ☐1 ☐2 |

_____

| **Fat** | 1,350-Calorie Plan ☐1 ☐2 ☐3 ☐4 | 1,600-Calorie Plan ☐5 ☐6 | 2,200-Calorie Plan ☐7 ☐8 |

_____

_____

| **Water** | All Plans ☐1 ☐2 ☐3 ☐4 ☐5 ☐6 ☐7 ☐8 |

_____

_____

PILATES

☐ I did a Pilates session today.   ☐ I did my warmup and cooldown stretches.

CARDIO EXERCISE

Type of cardio I did today: _____

Minutes of cardio I did today: _____ Day of my next cardio session: _____

POSITIVE THINKING

Positive-thinking exercise I did today: _____ ☐ I made time for me today.

How I felt about myself today: _____

How I can feel even better tomorrow: _____

RESULTS

Changes I see so far today (lengthening, toning, and so forth): _____

_____

Changes I feel so far (strengthening, energy levels, mental outlook, and so forth): _____

_____

Other improvements: _____

_____

Additional thoughts: _____

_____

Day 11 MY EATING PLAN

Food	Daily Servings			Healthiest foods I selected today:

Fruits and Vegetables

1,350-Calorie Plan	1,600-Calorie Plan	2,200-Calorie Plan
☐1 ☐2 ☐3 ☐4 ☐5	☐6 ☐7	☐8 ☐9

Whole Grains

1,350- and 1,600-Calorie Plans	2,200-Calorie Plan
☐1 ☐2 ☐3 ☐4 ☐5 ☐6	☐7 ☐8 ☐9

Starch

1,350-Calorie Plan	1,600-Calorie Plan	2,200-Calorie Plan
☐1	☐2	☐3

Protein — All Plans ☐1 ☐2

Dairy — All Plans ☐1 ☐2

Fat

1,350-Calorie Plan	1,600-Calorie Plan	2,200-Calorie Plan
☐1 ☐2 ☐3 ☐4	☐5 ☐6	☐7 ☐8

Water — All Plans ☐1 ☐2 ☐3 ☐4 ☐5 ☐6 ☐7 ☐8

Healthiest foods I selected today:

_____

_____

_____

_____

How I can improve tomorrow:

_____

_____

_____

_____

_____

_____

PILATES

☐ I did a Pilates session today.   ☐ I did my warmup and cooldown stretches.

CARDIO EXERCISE

Type of cardio I did today: _____

Minutes of cardio I did today: _____ Day of my next cardio session: _____

POSITIVE THINKING

Positive-thinking exercise I did today: _____ ☐ I made time for me today.

How I felt about myself today: _____

How I can feel even better tomorrow: _____

RESULTS

Changes I see so far today (lengthening, toning, and so forth): _____

_____

Changes I feel so far (strengthening, energy levels, mental outlook, and so forth): _____

_____

Other improvements: _____

_____

Additional thoughts: _____

_____

Day 12 MY EATING PLAN

Food	Daily Servings			Healthiest foods I selected today:
Fruits and Vegetables	**1,350-Calorie Plan** ☐ 1 ☐ 2 ☐ 3 ☐ 4 ☐ 5	**1,600-Calorie Plan** ☐ 6 ☐ 7	**2,200-Calorie Plan** ☐ 8 ☐ 9	
Whole Grains	**1,350- and 1,600-Calorie Plans** ☐ 1 ☐ 2 ☐ 3 ☐ 4 ☐ 5 ☐ 6		**2,200-Calorie Plan** ☐ 7 ☐ 8 ☐ 9	
Starch	**1,350-Calorie Plan** ☐ 1	**1,600-Calorie Plan** ☐ 2	**2,200-Calorie Plan** ☐ 3	
Protein	All Plans ☐ 1 ☐ 2			How I can improve tomorrow:
Dairy	All Plans ☐ 1 ☐ 2			
Fat	**1,350-Calorie Plan** ☐ 1 ☐ 2 ☐ 3 ☐ 4	**1,600-Calorie Plan** ☐ 5 ☐ 6	**2,200-Calorie Plan** ☐ 7 ☐ 8	
Water	All Plans ☐ 1 ☐ 2 ☐ 3 ☐ 4 ☐ 5 ☐ 6 ☐ 7 ☐ 8			

PILATES

☐ I did a Pilates session today.   ☐ I did my warmup and cooldown stretches.

CARDIO EXERCISE

Type of cardio I did today: _____

Minutes of cardio I did today: _____   Day of my next cardio session: _____

POSITIVE THINKING

Positive-thinking exercise I did today: _____   ☐ I made time for me today.

How I felt about myself today: _____

How I can feel even better tomorrow: _____

RESULTS

Changes I see so far today (lengthening, toning, and so forth): _____

_____

Changes I feel so far (strengthening, energy levels, mental outlook, and so forth): _____

_____

Other improvements: _____

_____

Additional thoughts: _____

_____

Day 13 MY EATING PLAN

Food	Daily Servings			Healthiest foods I selected today:

Fruits and Vegetables

1,350-Calorie Plan	1,600-Calorie Plan	2,200-Calorie Plan
☐1 ☐2 ☐3 ☐4 ☐5	☐6 ☐7	☐8 ☐9

Whole Grains

1,350- and 1,600-Calorie Plans	2,200-Calorie Plan
☐1 ☐2 ☐3 ☐4 ☐5 ☐6	☐7 ☐8 ☐9

Starch

1,350-Calorie Plan	1,600-Calorie Plan	2,200-Calorie Plan
☐1	☐2	☐3

Protein   All Plans ☐1 ☐2

Dairy   All Plans ☐1 ☐2

Fat

1,350-Calorie Plan	1,600-Calorie Plan	2,200-Calorie Plan
☐1 ☐2 ☐3 ☐4	☐5 ☐6	☐7 ☐8

Water   All Plans ☐1 ☐2 ☐3 ☐4 ☐5 ☐6 ☐7 ☐8

Healthiest foods I selected today:
_____
_____
_____
_____

How I can improve tomorrow:
_____
_____
_____
_____
_____
_____

PILATES

☐ I did a Pilates session today.   ☐ I did my warmup and cooldown stretches.

CARDIO EXERCISE

Type of cardio I did today: _____

Minutes of cardio I did today: _____ Day of my next cardio session: _____

POSITIVE THINKING

Positive-thinking exercise I did today: _____ ☐ I made time for me today.

How I felt about myself today: _____

How I can feel even better tomorrow: _____

RESULTS

Changes I see so far today (lengthening, toning, and so forth): _____

_____

Changes I feel so far (strengthening, energy levels, mental outlook, and so forth): _____

_____

Other improvements: _____

_____

Additional thoughts: _____

_____

Day 14 MY EATING PLAN

Food	Daily Servings		
Fruits and Vegetables	1,350-Calorie Plan ☐ 1 ☐ 2 ☐ 3 ☐ 4 ☐ 5	1,600-Calorie Plan ☐ 6 ☐ 7	2,200-Calorie Plan ☐ 8 ☐ 9
Whole Grains	1,350- and 1,600-Calorie Plans ☐ 1 ☐ 2 ☐ 3 ☐ 4 ☐ 5 ☐ 6		2,200-Calorie Plan ☐ 7 ☐ 8 ☐ 9
Starch	1,350-Calorie Plan ☐ 1	1,600-Calorie Plan ☐ 2	2,200-Calorie Plan ☐ 3
Protein	All Plans ☐ 1 ☐ 2		
Dairy	All Plans ☐ 1 ☐ 2		
Fat	1,350-Calorie Plan ☐ 1 ☐ 2 ☐ 3 ☐ 4	1,600-Calorie Plan ☐ 5 ☐ 6	2,200-Calorie Plan ☐ 7 ☐ 8
Water	All Plans ☐ 1 ☐ 2 ☐ 3 ☐ 4 ☐ 5 ☐ 6 ☐ 7 ☐ 8		

Healthiest foods I selected today:

_____

_____

_____

_____

How I can improve tomorrow:

_____

_____

_____

_____

_____

PILATES

☐ I did a Pilates session today.　　☐ I did my warmup and cooldown stretches.

CARDIO EXERCISE

Type of cardio I did today: _____

Minutes of cardio I did today: _____　Day of my next cardio session: _____

POSITIVE THINKING

Positive-thinking exercise I did today: _____　☐ I made time for me today.

How I felt about myself today: _____

How I can feel even better tomorrow: _____

RESULTS

Changes I see so far today (lengthening, toning, and so forth): _____

_____

Changes I feel so far (strengthening, energy levels, mental outlook, and so forth): _____

_____

Other improvements: _____

_____

Additional thoughts: _____

_____

Day 15 MY EATING PLAN

Food	Daily Servings		
Fruits and Vegetables	1,350-Calorie Plan ☐ 1 ☐ 2 ☐ 3 ☐ 4 ☐ 5	1,600-Calorie Plan ☐ 6 ☐ 7	2,200-Calorie Plan ☐ 8 ☐ 9
Whole Grains	1,350- and 1,600-Calorie Plans ☐ 1 ☐ 2 ☐ 3 ☐ 4 ☐ 5 ☐ 6		2,200-Calorie Plan ☐ 7 ☐ 8 ☐ 9
Starch	1,350-Calorie Plan ☐ 1	1,600-Calorie Plan ☐ 2	2,200-Calorie Plan ☐ 3
Protein	All Plans ☐ 1 ☐ 2		
Dairy	All Plans ☐ 1 ☐ 2		
Fat	1,350-Calorie Plan ☐ 1 ☐ 2 ☐ 3 ☐ 4	1,600-Calorie Plan ☐ 5 ☐ 6	2,200-Calorie Plan ☐ 7 ☐ 8
Water	All Plans ☐ 1 ☐ 2 ☐ 3 ☐ 4 ☐ 5 ☐ 6 ☐ 7 ☐ 8		

Healthiest foods I selected today:

_____

_____

_____

_____

How I can improve tomorrow:

_____

_____

_____

_____

_____

PILATES

☐ I did a Pilates session today.   ☐ I did my warmup and cooldown stretches.

CARDIO EXERCISE

Type of cardio I did today: _____

Minutes of cardio I did today: _____ Day of my next cardio session: _____

POSITIVE THINKING

Positive-thinking exercise I did today: _____ ☐ I made time for me today.

How I felt about myself today: _____

How I can feel even better tomorrow: _____

RESULTS

Changes I see so far today (lengthening, toning, and so forth): _____

_____

Changes I feel so far (strengthening, energy levels, mental outlook, and so forth): _____

_____

Other improvements: _____

_____

Additional thoughts: _____

_____

Day 16 MY EATING PLAN

Food	Daily Servings		
Fruits and Vegetables	1,350-Calorie Plan ☐1 ☐2 ☐3 ☐4 ☐5	1,600-Calorie Plan ☐6 ☐7	2,200-Calorie Plan ☐8 ☐9
Whole Grains	1,350- and 1,600-Calorie Plans ☐1 ☐2 ☐3 ☐4 ☐5 ☐6		2,200-Calorie Plan ☐7 ☐8 ☐9
Starch	1,350-Calorie Plan ☐1	1,600-Calorie Plan ☐2	2,200-Calorie Plan ☐3
Protein	All Plans ☐1 ☐2		
Dairy	All Plans ☐1 ☐2		
Fat	1,350-Calorie Plan ☐1 ☐2 ☐3 ☐4	1,600-Calorie Plan ☐5 ☐6	2,200-Calorie Plan ☐7 ☐8
Water	All Plans ☐1 ☐2 ☐3 ☐4 ☐5 ☐6 ☐7 ☐8		

Healthiest foods I selected today:

_____
_____
_____
_____

How I can improve tomorrow:

_____
_____
_____
_____
_____
_____

PILATES

☐ I did a Pilates session today.   ☐ I did my warmup and cooldown stretches.

CARDIO EXERCISE

Type of cardio I did today: _____

Minutes of cardio I did today: _____ Day of my next cardio session: _____

POSITIVE THINKING

Positive-thinking exercise I did today: _____ ☐ I made time for me today.

How I felt about myself today: _____

How I can feel even better tomorrow: _____

RESULTS

Changes I see so far today (lengthening, toning, and so forth): _____

_____

Changes I feel so far (strengthening, energy levels, mental outlook, and so forth): _____

_____

Other improvements: _____

_____

Additional thoughts: _____

_____

Day 17 MY EATING PLAN

Food	Daily Servings			Healthiest foods I selected today:

Fruits and Vegetables

1,350-Calorie Plan	1,600-Calorie Plan	2,200-Calorie Plan
☐1 ☐2 ☐3 ☐4 ☐5	☐6 ☐7	☐8 ☐9

_____
_____
_____
_____

Whole Grains

1,350- and 1,600-Calorie Plans	2,200-Calorie Plan
☐1 ☐2 ☐3 ☐4 ☐5 ☐6	☐7 ☐8 ☐9

Starch

1,350-Calorie Plan	1,600-Calorie Plan	2,200-Calorie Plan
☐1	☐2	☐3

How I can improve tomorrow:

Protein All Plans ☐1 ☐2

Dairy All Plans ☐1 ☐2

_____
_____

Fat

1,350-Calorie Plan	1,600-Calorie Plan	2,200-Calorie Plan
☐1 ☐2 ☐3 ☐4	☐5 ☐6	☐7 ☐8

Water All Plans ☐1 ☐2 ☐3 ☐4 ☐5 ☐6 ☐7 ☐8

_____
_____
_____

PILATES

☐ I did a Pilates session today.   ☐ I did my warmup and cooldown stretches.

CARDIO EXERCISE

Type of cardio I did today: _____

Minutes of cardio I did today: _____ Day of my next cardio session: _____

POSITIVE THINKING

Positive-thinking exercise I did today: _____ ☐ I made time for me today.

How I felt about myself today: _____

How I can feel even better tomorrow: _____

RESULTS

Changes I see so far today (lengthening, toning, and so forth): _____

_____

Changes I feel so far (strengthening, energy levels, mental outlook, and so forth): _____

_____

Other improvements: _____

_____

Additional thoughts: _____

_____

Day 18 MY EATING PLAN

Food	Daily Servings			Healthiest foods I selected today:

Fruits and Vegetables

1,350-Calorie Plan	1,600-Calorie Plan	2,200-Calorie Plan
☐1 ☐2 ☐3 ☐4 ☐5	☐6 ☐7	☐8 ☐9

Whole Grains

1,350- and 1,600-Calorie Plans	2,200-Calorie Plan
☐1 ☐2 ☐3 ☐4 ☐5 ☐6	☐7 ☐8 ☐9

Starch

1,350-Calorie Plan	1,600-Calorie Plan	2,200-Calorie Plan
☐1	☐2	☐3

Protein All Plans ☐1 ☐2

Dairy All Plans ☐1 ☐2

Fat

1,350-Calorie Plan	1,600-Calorie Plan	2,200-Calorie Plan
☐1 ☐2 ☐3 ☐4	☐5 ☐6	☐7 ☐8

Water All Plans ☐1 ☐2 ☐3 ☐4 ☐5 ☐6 ☐7 ☐8

Healthiest foods I selected today:

_____

_____

_____

_____

How I can improve tomorrow:

_____

_____

_____

_____

_____

_____

PILATES

☐ I did a Pilates session today. ☐ I did my warmup and cooldown stretches.

CARDIO EXERCISE

Type of cardio I did today: _____

Minutes of cardio I did today: _____ Day of my next cardio session: _____

POSITIVE THINKING

Positive-thinking exercise I did today: _____ ☐ I made time for me today.

How I felt about myself today: _____

How I can feel even better tomorrow: _____

RESULTS

Changes I see so far today (lengthening, toning, and so forth): _____

_____

Changes I feel so far (strengthening, energy levels, mental outlook, and so forth): _____

_____

Other improvements: _____

_____

Additional thoughts: _____

_____

Day 19 MY EATING PLAN

Food	Daily Servings			Healthiest foods I selected today:
Fruits and Vegetables	1,350-Calorie Plan ☐1 ☐2 ☐3 ☐4 ☐5	1,600-Calorie Plan ☐6 ☐7	2,200-Calorie Plan ☐8 ☐9	
Whole Grains	1,350- and 1,600-Calorie Plans ☐1 ☐2 ☐3 ☐4 ☐5 ☐6		2,200-Calorie Plan ☐7 ☐8 ☐9	
Starch	1,350-Calorie Plan ☐1	1,600-Calorie Plan ☐2	2,200-Calorie Plan ☐3	
Protein	All Plans ☐1 ☐2			
Dairy	All Plans ☐1 ☐2			
Fat	1,350-Calorie Plan ☐1 ☐2 ☐3 ☐4	1,600-Calorie Plan ☐5 ☐6	2,200-Calorie Plan ☐7 ☐8	
Water	All Plans ☐1 ☐2 ☐3 ☐4 ☐5 ☐6 ☐7 ☐8			

Healthiest foods I selected today:

_____

_____

_____

How I can improve tomorrow:

_____

_____

_____

_____

_____

_____

PILATES

☐ I did a Pilates session today.   ☐ I did my warmup and cooldown stretches.

CARDIO EXERCISE

Type of cardio I did today: _____

Minutes of cardio I did today: _____ Day of my next cardio session: _____

POSITIVE THINKING

Positive-thinking exercise I did today: _____ ☐ I made time for me today.

How I felt about myself today: _____

How I can feel even better tomorrow: _____

RESULTS

Changes I see so far today (lengthening, toning, and so forth): _____

_____

Changes I feel so far (strengthening, energy levels, mental outlook, and so forth): _____

_____

Other improvements: _____

_____

Additional thoughts: _____

_____

Day 20   MY EATING PLAN

Food	Daily Servings		
Fruits and Vegetables	**1,350-Calorie Plan** ☐1 ☐2 ☐3 ☐4 ☐5	**1,600-Calorie Plan** ☐6 ☐7	**2,200-Calorie Plan** ☐8 ☐9
Whole Grains	**1,350- and 1,600-Calorie Plans** ☐1 ☐2 ☐3 ☐4 ☐5 ☐6		**2,200-Calorie Plan** ☐7 ☐8 ☐9
Starch	**1,350-Calorie Plan** ☐1	**1,600-Calorie Plan** ☐2	**2,200-Calorie Plan** ☐3
Protein	All Plans ☐1 ☐2		
Dairy	All Plans ☐1 ☐2		
Fat	**1,350-Calorie Plan** ☐1 ☐2 ☐3 ☐4	**1,600-Calorie Plan** ☐5 ☐6	**2,200-Calorie Plan** ☐7 ☐8
Water	All Plans ☐1 ☐2 ☐3 ☐4 ☐5 ☐6 ☐7 ☐8		

Healthiest foods I selected today:

_____

_____

_____

_____

How I can improve tomorrow:

_____

_____

_____

_____

_____

PILATES

☐ I did a Pilates session today.   ☐ I did my warmup and cooldown stretches.

CARDIO EXERCISE

Type of cardio I did today: _____

Minutes of cardio I did today: _____ Day of my next cardio session: _____

POSITIVE THINKING

Positive-thinking exercise I did today: _____ ☐ I made time for me today.

How I felt about myself today: _____

How I can feel even better tomorrow: _____

RESULTS

Changes I see so far today (lengthening, toning, and so forth): _____

_____

Changes I feel so far (strengthening, energy levels, mental outlook, and so forth): _____

_____

Other improvements: _____

_____

Additional thoughts: _____

_____

Day

MY EATING PLAN

Food	Daily Servings			Healthiest foods I selected today:

Fruits and Vegetables	**1,350-Calorie Plan** ☐1 ☐2 ☐3 ☐4 ☐5	**1,600-Calorie Plan** ☐6 ☐7	**2,200-Calorie Plan** ☐8 ☐9

Healthiest foods I selected today:
_____
_____
_____
_____

Whole Grains	**1,350- and 1,600-Calorie Plans** ☐1 ☐2 ☐3 ☐4 ☐5 ☐6	**2,200-Calorie Plan** ☐7 ☐8 ☐9

Starch	**1,350-Calorie Plan** ☐1	**1,600-Calorie Plan** ☐2	**2,200-Calorie Plan** ☐3

How I can improve tomorrow:
_____
_____

Protein	All Plans ☐1 ☐2

Dairy	All Plans ☐1 ☐2

Fat	**1,350-Calorie Plan** ☐1 ☐2 ☐3 ☐4	**1,600-Calorie Plan** ☐5 ☐6	**2,200-Calorie Plan** ☐7 ☐8

Water	All Plans ☐1 ☐2 ☐3 ☐4 ☐5 ☐6 ☐7 ☐8

_____
_____
_____
_____

PILATES

☐ I did a Pilates session today.   ☐ I did my warmup and cooldown stretches.

CARDIO EXERCISE

Type of cardio I did today: _____

Minutes of cardio I did today: _____ Day of my next cardio session: _____

POSITIVE THINKING

Positive-thinking exercise I did today: _____ ☐ I made time for me today.

How I felt about myself today: _____

How I can feel even better tomorrow: _____

RESULTS

Changes I see so far today (lengthening, toning, and so forth): _____
_____

Changes I feel so far (strengthening, energy levels, mental outlook, and so forth): _____
_____

Other improvements: _____
_____

Additional thoughts: _____
_____

Index

Underscored page references indicate sidebars and tables. **Boldface** references indicate photographs and illustrations.

299

o

Obliques, Pilates targeting, 7, **7**, 173
Oblique strengthener
   in 10-Minute Advanced Abdominal Routine, 182, **182**
   in 3-Week Pilates Program, **272**
Oblique strengthener with towel, in 10-Minute Healthy Back Routine, 191–92, **191–92**
Obstacles to exercise, overcoming, 248
Oils, healthy choices of, 224
Olive oil, 224
Olives, monounsaturated fats in, 224
Omega-3 fatty acids
   health benefits from, 217
   sources of, 223, 224
One-leg lift
   in Beginner Pilates Program, 42, **42**, **61**
   in 3-Week Pilates Program, **255**
Open leg stretch, as yoga cooldown in 3-Week Pilates Program, 265, **265**
Osteoarthritis. *See* Arthritis
Outer hip and thigh slimmer, in 5-Minute Balance Ball Routine, 205, **205**
Overhead press
   in 10-Minute Upper Body Routine, 171, **171**
   in 3-Week Pilates Program, **272**
Overweight, workouts suitable with, 30, 35

p

Pain
   Pilates relieving, 12, 13–14
   workouts suitable with, 30, 35, 137
Partially hydrogenated oil, avoiding, 217, 224
Peanut butter, monounsaturated fats in, 224
Percussion breathing, 33, 173
Perfect ab curl, in 10-Minute Healthy Back Routine, 194, **194**
Pilates, Joseph H., 3, 4–5, 8, 29
Pilates for Every Body book
   how to use, 23–25
   overview of exercises in, 4
   Pilates Pointers in, 21, 32
Pilates for Every Body video, 5, 13, 24, 24, 31
Pilates Pointer of the Week
   purpose of, 252
   for week 1 of 3-Week Pilates Program, 254

for week 3 of 3-Week Pilates Program, 269
for week 2 of 3-Week Pilates Program, 261
Pilates Pointers in this book, purpose of, 21, 32
Pilates pushup
   in Complete Pilates Program, 103–4, **103–4**, **118**
   in 3-Week Pilates Program, **266**, **275**
Plank
   in 10-Minute Advanced Abdominal Routine, 179–80, **179–80**
   in 3-Week Pilates Program, **266**
Plié
   in 10-Minute Hip, Thigh, and Butt Routine, 144, **144**
   in 3-Week Pilates Program, **257**
Portion sizes, in eating plan, 226–27
Positive feedback on Pilates, 9–12
Positive-thinking program
   benefits from, 247
   overview of, 212
   techniques in, 248–51
Postpregnancy exercise, workouts suitable for, 30, 35
Posture
   Pilates improving, 14, **14**
   pointers for, in Pilates, **17–19**
Powerhouse
   as key to Pilates, 6–8
   posture and, **14**
   in upper body routine, 161
Power Yoga Plus video, 10, 24, 31
Precision, as Pilates principle, 21
Pregnancy
   abdominal toning after, 11–12, 15, 187
   back pain during, 186
   workouts suitable after, 137
Principles of Pilates, 19–22
Progressive Pilates, overview of, 212. *See also* 3-Week Pilates Program
Proteins, in eating plan, 222–23
   serving sizes of, 227
Punches, in in-home cardio routine, 246
Pushup, in 5-Minute Balance Ball Routine, 203, **203**
Pushup, Pilates
   in Complete Pilates Program, 103–4, **103–4**, **118**
   in 3-Week Pilates Program, **266**, **275**